Regulating British M
The General Medical Council

Regulating British Medicine: The General Medical Council

MARGARET STACEY
Emeritus Professor, University of Warwick, UK

JOHN WILEY & SONS
Chichester · New York · Brisbane · Toronto · Singapore

Other Wiley Editorial Offices

John Wiley & Sons, Inc., 605 Third Avenue,
New York, NY 10158–0012, USA

Jacaranda Wiley Ltd, G.P.O. Box 859, Brisbane,
Queensland 4001, Australia

John Wiley & Sons (Canada) Ltd, 22 Worcester Road,
Rexdale, Ontario M9W 1L1, Canada

John Wiley & Sons (SEA) Pte Ltd, 37 Jalan Pemimpin # 05-04,
Block B, Union Industrial Building, Singapore 2057

Library of Congress Cataloging-in-Publication Data

Stacey, Margaret.
    Regulating British medicine : the General Medical Council /
Margaret Stacey.
        p. cm.
    Includes bibliographical references and index.
    ISBN 0-471-93189-6
    1. General Medical Council (Great Britain) 2. Medicine, State—
Great Britain. I. Title.
    [DNLM: 1. General Medical Council (Great Britain) 2. State
Medicine—organization & administration—Great Britain. 3. State
Medicine—trends—Great Britain. W 275 FA1 S77r]
RA241.S83 1992
362.1′0941—dc20
DNLM/DLC
for Library of Congress   92-5579
                                                                        CIP

British Library Cataloguing in Publication Data

A catalogue record for this book is
available from the British Library

ISBN 0 471 93189 6

Typeset in 10/12 pt Palacio by Mathematical Composition Setters Ltd, Salisbury
Printed in Great Britain by Biddles Ltd, Guildford

This book is dedicated to all those practitioners for whom healing the sick and alleviating suffering is their prime goal

Contents

List of Tables

List of Figures

Acknowledgements

There are many people whose help in the production of this book I must acknowledge. The ESRC gave me the grant (G00232247) which made the work possible. Judy Morris helped with data analysis and many (often tedious) secretarial and clerical tasks. All of these she undertook with exemplary thoroughness. Thanks for secretarial help must also go to Eileen Clark. While not ever directly employed on this research, successive sociology department secretaries have for many years provided friendly help and support for which many thanks.

Without the co-operation of the Presidents of the GMC, past and present, Lord Richardson, Lord Walton and Sir Robert Kilpatrick, this work would not have been possible. They offered help and support and spared valuable time to talk to me notwithstanding that they recognized in me a critical ex-member: my gratitude to them. Many past and present members of the Council, both medical and lay, also spared valuable time to talk to me: for that I am immensely grateful, as I am to other doctors and 'lay' persons knowledgeable about the Council who also gave me of their time. To those who read and critically commented on draft papers, my debt is even greater.

Members of the Warwick University Department of Sociology and the Medical Sociology Group of the British Sociological Association afforded me valuble space to present portions of the material in seminars and at meetings. Their friendly critical comment was most valuable. My thanks to them.

My gratitude also to Sarida Brown for helping me overcome some of the personal dilemmas the research presented me with. Jennifer Lorch has earned special thanks for the love and loyalty she has offered throughout the many vicissitudes I encountered in bringing this book to completion.

I am grateful to David Gullick for permission to use material from his article 'The General Medical Council Steeplechase' and to Jean Scott and *The British Medical Journal* for permission to use data from her article 'Women and the GMC'.

Without access to the many official publications of the GMC itself, this book could not have been written. However, my use of these documents does not imply the Council's endorsement or approval of the book's contents, or that the book reflects the views or opinions of the Council or of its past or present members.

Notwithstanding all the debts I owe to so many people, named and unnamed, and which I gratefully acknowledge, only I am responsible for any errors or omissions there may be in this book and for the opinions expressed therein.

Note When occasionally 'we' is used in this book it is to stand for 'you, the reader and I'.

PART 1
INTRODUCTION

1

Origins and Nature of the Research

This book is offered as a contribution to the debate about the regulation of the medical profession—a debate which has been on the agenda of patients' organizations for many years, but which in its present form has been precipitated by government, beginning with the Monopolies Commission Report, the restrictive practices white paper (Cm. 331) and the NHS Review (Cm. 555). Standards of ethics and of competence are of prime interest to medical practitioners and patients alike. All our futures may be affected by the outcome of the debates. I believe it is crucial for the common good that these debates should be open to a wide variety of interests and be as well-informed as possible.

It has been a difficult book to write. I have found so much that is right and so much that is wrong about the General Medical Council (GMC). Later on I shall explain what I mean by right and wrong in this context—right or wrong in what terms and whose terms. First, however, let me explain how it has come about that I, a lay person, should be writing the book at all.

I came to the GMC as a lay member in 1976 and served until 1984. Before that I had served on a Welsh Hospital Management Committee and then on the Welsh Hospital Board until its dissolution in 1974. Along the way I had been a member of the Michael Davies Committee on Hospital Complaints Procedures. My route to those bodies had begun with a concern about the welfare of children in hospital.

The circumspect enquiry which came over the telephone one day as to whether I would accept membership of the GMC if asked left me with a sense of awe—as well as surprise and wonder. As I wrote some time ago:

Before I became a member, the General Medical Council had always seemed to me to be a somewhat shadowy body. I recall during the difficulties of 1972 seeing a newspaper picture of grey haired and balding men leaving the

> Council building; the implication was that no one would be surprised to learn that such an elderly group, unrepresentative of their profession, were out of touch and had trouble on their hands. Little did I imagine then that in 1975 [I should have written 1976 as I now know] I would be summoned to serve and would become one of them (also elderly and grey haired, but neither a doctor nor a man).
>
> *GMC Annual Report for 1983*, p. 21

I accepted the Privy Council nomination in a spirit of public service. In accepting office I was aware that I preferred policy-making work to regulatory work, but accepted the 'calling' nevertheless.

From the outset it occurred to me that I might wish to inform the lay public about how the GMC, a somewhat mysterious body, actually worked. What I had in mind was advice to patients' organizations, for example. To this end, before accepting nomination I enquired whether it would be permitted to talk or write about the Council. I was assured that it would be, so long as the Council could check any writing before publication 'as to matters of fact'. This request I have complied with in anything I have written about the Council—including this book. When I first sat on the Council, however, it did not at once occur to me that I might one day undertake formal research. That thought came later.

As the years went by I became intrigued by, but also worried about, the workings of the GMC. Various people, interested in professional regulation or the handling of consumer complaints, pressed me to write up what I knew of the Council. Two things held me back. One was that as a trained researcher I had qualms about 'shooting off my mouth' without looking at the evidence systematically. The other was that a full-time teaching post and administrative responsibilities in the university, with public office added, left little time for any writing, let alone research.

There are, I suppose, two main sorts of accounts which are written by people who have been closely involved in a public institution. One is the officially commissioned history, which generally tends to take the form of an apologia and to be of limited use to future researchers—although of great encouragement to the faithful. The other is memoirs. Such works can also be informative but may well tell more about the author than the institution. As the first sociologist on the GMC, I thought perhaps I could give an account which would be of interest not only to lay people but also to medical practitioners themselves, for I knew they were and are most anxious to regulate their profession well.

Consequently I applied for research funds, not for a research assistant but for time off to do the research myself with the help of a research secretary. The first application failed. The second, to the Economic and Social Research Council (ESRC), succeeded.

The aim of the research, which the ESRC funded (grant number G00 232247), was to do a sociological analysis of the Council for the period from 1976 to 1984, the time during which I was a lay member. The committee of inquiry into the regulation of the medical profession, chaired by Sir Alec Merrison, had started work in 1973 and reported in 1975; the Act which was to reform the Council was passed in 1978. I served for the last session of the old Council and for the first session of the new.

This was a critical period for other reasons as well. After 1979 government began to give encouragement to private practice, encouragement renewed in the 1989 NHS Review (Cm. 555) and the 1990 NHS Act. This increase in private practice refreshed concern about advertising and anxiety about responsibility for regulating practice which fell outside the NHS complaints procedures. Also during this period the EC directives about labour mobility and harmonization as they applied to medicine became operative. No longer was the GMC the sovereign authority on who should have the right to practise medicine in the UK. Finally, throughout the period the voice of the patient and the potential patient, increasingly heard since the Second World War, became louder; mass media, while dramatizing the contributions of high-technology medicine, also subjected the medical profession to considerable criticism.

In order to research that period properly it was, of course, necessary to look at the antecedents of those historic changes of the 1970s. Naturally, also, I have tried to follow up what has happened since I left the Council, especially in terms of developments which were already afoot before 1984. My evaluation of the earlier and later periods obviously lacks the insights from personal involvement which I can bring to bear on the events of 1976–1984.

From the outset in planning the research I had the support of the Council's then president, Sir John Walton, and very full co-operation from Mr Peter Towers, the registrar. Sir Robert Kilpatrick, the present president elected in 1989, is equally helpful. Lord Richardson, who was president when I was first appointed to the Council and throughout the period between the Merrison Report and the establishment of the reconstituted Council, has also offered his full co-operation, as has Mr Martin Draper, the former registrar. At the outset I wrote to all those members of the Council who served during the period when I was a member, as well as to all those who were serving when my research began, to tell them what I was trying to do. I was greatly heartened by the very many warm letters which I received in response and by the willingness of members to be interviewed. I have personally interviewed 30 members and others in connection with the research and am most grateful to them all and to those who have responded to written enquiries.

The focus of my research has been on the tensions the Council experiences between maintaining the unity of the profession on the one hand and protecting the public on the other, the latter being a statutory charge which is laid upon it. The ability of the Council to regulate the profession depends on the latter remaining united, retaining confidence in the Council and accepting its legitimacy to control the profession. This was nearly lost in 1968–1973 (see Chapter 3).

I isolated the following themes to pursue in greater detail: professional unity versus public responsibility; clinical autonomy versus competence to practise; control of educational standards; the GMC and the DHSS (as it then was); the GMC and the profession. I left space in my plans to pursue other themes which might emerge. The whole exercise was really to be a study of the way medical professional self-regulation worked in practice during my period of service on the Council. What I am now doing is using that research as a jumping-off ground for a more general review of the Council as a crucial part of medical self-regulation at this time when profound changes are in the air. More detailed and 'academic' accounts of particular aspects of the period I have studied have been or will be prepared for learned journals.

From participant to observer

The research is of course somewhat unusual—even for social science research—in that I was a participant before I became a scientific observer. As I have said, I did not join the Council for research purposes as a participant observer, but as a public representative appointed by the Privy Council. As a lay member I felt it my responsibility to speak on behalf of the public and to interpret popular views of the Council and the medical profession to the medical members. As a social scientist I had an interest in the Council's attitude to the social sciences in medical education. As a woman I expressed interest in those issues which concern women doctors (a small minority of the Council's membership) and also in the treatment of women as patients. Opposed to racial discrimination, I paid attention to the problems of overseas doctors and to the recognition of medical schools overseas.

So over the nine years I was a committed participant who took certain political stances (in a non-party sense). Notwithstanding this I always felt somewhat marginal to the proceedings, a marginality stemming from my womanhood (sometimes being the only woman on a committee, sometimes one of two) and from my lay status. While I came to share with medical members a feeling for the work of the Council I could never fully participate in their shared medical culture derived from a common medical education and practice experiences. Nor did I share their material interests, earning my living in other ways than theirs. Nevertheless in that context (and informed by 20 years of research in medical sociology) I probably came as near to understanding medical culture and structure as it is possible for a lay woman to do. My background in medical sociology ensured that I did not, as some lay members do, become 'more medical than the medical'.

My involvement was not just the twice-yearly Council meetings: I served on the education committee throughout my two terms of office; on the disciplinary committee and later on the newly established health committee; in the second session I was also on the executive committee. But I was never so near the heart of the matter as to be on finance and establishment; lay members did not serve on that committee in my day, although one now does (1991). After a year's self-imposed reticence, I spoke out, especially on the topics I have mentioned.

Attempting to gain detachment

When it came to doing the research, I felt that I needed someone to help me, not only because of the amount of work to do, but also to help me get the distance I would need. Hence the request for a research secretary and the subsequent appointment of Judy Morris, a graduate. Her task was to make and keep records and chase references as well as carry out all the regular secretarial duties and to point out to me if she came across evidence that I was misinterpreting data. It was she who indicated to me that I was appointed in 1976 and not 1975 as I had written in the GMC annual report. When she left, which was not before she had completed the major data extraction tasks she had been set, she was succeeded by Eileen Clark.

When I went on the Council, members had access to transcripts of any proceedings they might want to look at. When discussing the research at the outset I had been told that, if I wished them, transcripts would be made available to me. There were two reasons why they would be useful: first, as a check on the accuracy of my memory or any notes that I had made at the time; and second, to read how I had behaved, thus getting a better idea of what my role and stance was. When it came to analysing disciplinary and health committee proceedings I particularly wanted to know whether I reacted on those committees as most other lay members do. However, during the period of my research there was a policy change (see Chapter 11) and I was not permitted to read any of the transcripts except for committees on which I had sat. It has therefore not been possible for me to make any comparison of my role—on disciplinary committees, for example—with that of other lay members.

The method I have had to rely upon to try and ensure some detachment in my account is to show working papers when I have written them to key members of Council so far as that topic is concerned. Members have been most helpful and frank in their criticisms and comments.

The sources which I have used have been the publicly available documents published by the GMC such as the annual reports, the minutes, published annually, the register, the confidential papers which I received as a member for meetings I attended (sometimes annotated), and a diary in which I noted what I thought was important in what had happened. I am not a good diarist; sometimes the diary was written that night, sometimes next morning, sometimes not until quite a long time after—and it has quite considerable gaps.

I have tried systematically to take aspects of the Council's work relevant to the central theme and trace them through the documents, paying attention to two aspects: how the issues are dealt with within Council and what is said in the medical and also to some extent the lay worlds about the Council's actions. Between us Judy Morris and I looked at key medical weeklies, covering the *British Medical Journal*, *The Lancet*, *World Medicine*, *Pulse*, and the journal of the Medical Women's Federation for the entire period. I have not sought access to any personal records held by the Council. The data we recorded on a PC about members were those publicly available—when and how they came on to the Council, what committees they served on or offices they held. Nor shall I reveal material which is in the confidential papers which I have, although that and my memory will aid me in interpreting the publicly available material which I shall write about. Where my own knowledge and the records available have been insufficient, I have sought guidance from more knowledgeable members and officers. To them go my thanks for their help.

The book which follows is in five parts. This first part introduces the Council, explaining why, contrary to the opinion of some doctors, the GMC is important and outlining the Council's historical development up to 1968. Part 2 relates to the 1970s, the decade of the profession, when the reform of the Council followed lines which doctors suggested (although obviously not all agreed with all of them). The revolt, which began in the late 1960s, of the rank and file against the Council is described, the problems of and with overseas doctors, the Merrison enquiry and the subsequent 1978 Medical Act, how the composition of the Council was changed. Part 3 seeks to describe the workings of the Council in as straightforward a way as possible, covering the composition of the Council and how it changed, how it is structured, with major chapters on the central work of the Council: education and registration; and the maintenance of conduct and competence. That part is followed by Part 4 where what might be called the patients' revolt which characterized the 1980s as the decade of the 'consumers' is described. Part 5 is a critical evaluation of the Council as presently constituted and functioning, asking whether it is appropriate for the regulation of medicine in the 1990s. This part makes some suggestions for the future, concluding with the need for a new professionalism.

2

What the GMC Does and Why it Matters

A number of doctors in general and hospital practice around the country appear somewhat contemptuous of the GMC. Some argue that it does not matter very much, seeing other medical bodies as having more significance in maintaining standards. Others disapprove of its disciplinary actions, thinking it does no more than harass hard-working and well-meaning doctors. As to the lay public, most hardly know the GMC exists; even the well educated when challenged cannot with any certainty distinguish the GMC from the BMA (British Medical Association); those lay people who have had dealings with the GMC tend to be cynical about its activities as a protector of the public against doctors who may have behaved improperly.

However, the GMC is of considerable importance, both to members of the medical profession and to the public. It is the supreme regulating body of medicine in the UK, it plays an important part in setting the standards and ethos of medicine (or holding them back, according to one's point of view). It it the statutory body with powers granted by Parliament to regulate the profession. The essence of its power lies in its control of the registers of those competent to practise, which it keeps and publishes. Medical practitioners experience this power in two ways: first, the GMC controls entry to the register by deciding what qualifications are necessary for registration; second, it can remove practitioners from the register temporarily or permanently when they are deemed to have become unfit to practise. From the point of view of the public the GMC matters because in general terms it determines, through the registers, the sort of practitioners who may treat us and, with regard to specific individuals, who is fit to continue to treat us. The GMC seeks to ensure that our trust in registered medical practitioners is justified by ensuring the educational standard of entry in the register is maintained, and by removing doctors who are unfit to practise (Merrison Report, 1975, paragraphs 1 and 2).

The Council exercises its powers by approving medical schools and examining complaints received or convictions reported which affect professional conduct or the physical or mental fitness of registered medical practitioners. As to its oversight of basic medical education, the Council may visit and inspect medical schools. However, so far as continuing competence to practise is concerned, the Council has no inspectorate; it has to rely upon convictions reported or complaints initiated from outside to learn of professional misconduct. Since the 1978 Medical Act the GMC has the added responsibility for co-ordinating all stages of medical education. The registers and the Council's educational responsibilities will be discussed in greater detail in Chapters 9 and 10 and its disciplinary powers in Chapters 11 and 12.

The GMC also matters to the public because, to some extent directly through its own influence, but more importantly through that of doctors registered by it, the Council influences state decisions about medical care. The GMC is responsible to the Privy Council in the sense that, within the provisions of the Act, details of the constitution and functioning of the Council are provided by order of Her Majesty in [Privy] Council. Appeals against judgements of the GMC are made to the Privy Council.

The Council is based on the principle of professional self-regulation, and is the main instrument of that mode of control. It was established to ensure the profession's side of 'the contract between public and profession, by which the public go to the profession for medical treatment because the profession has made sure that it will provide satisfactory treatment' (Merrison Report, para. 4). Professional self-regulation in its turn is based upon the doctrine of clinical autonomy. This doctrine holds that a doctor is responsible only to his patient for diagnosis and treatment, and that only peers can comment on clinical judgements. The doctrine was perhaps most clearly stated in the 1974 debate on the reorganization of the NHS where the medical profession succeeded in enshrining the principle in the 'Grey Book' which constituted the bible of the 1974 NHS reorganization:

> The management arrangements required for the NHS are different from those commonly used in other large organizations because the work is different. The distinguishing characteristic of the NHS is that to do their work properly, consultants and general practitioners must have clinical autonomy, so that they can be fully responsible for the treatment they prescribe for their patients. It follows that these doctors and dentists work as each others' equals and that they are their own managers. In ethics and in law they are accountable to their patients for the care they prescribe, and they cannot be held accountable to the NHS authorities for the quality of their clinical judgements so long as they act within the broad limits of acceptable medical practice and within policy for the use of resources.
>
> DHSS (1972), 1.18

Insisting on this principle of clinical autonomy in 1974, the profession at that time avoided the managerial control which was imposed upon all other health care occupations and professions in the NHS.

It is because of the principle of professional self-regulation and the doctrine of clinical autonomy that the Council is essentially a professional body. In 1983 it was composed of 83 medical members and 7 lay members; the number of lay members has since been increased to 11 (see Chapter 7).

By statute the GMC is independent of the government and the NHS; it is funded directly by the practitioners themselves—although fees may be reclaimed as expenses or through tax relief. Nevertheless. the GMC is, by virtue of its statutory position, part of the apparatus of the central state. Members of the medical profession are not in constant consultation with cabinet ministers and senior civil servants, except when major health issues are involved—the threat of AIDS, for example, elevated the Chief Medical Officer (CMO) to the position of a cabinet adviser, a status formerly only accorded in wartime. It follows that GMC members constitute a relatively small part of the governing elite of this country, with regard to both the size and the importance of their presence. The more weight which is given nationally to health matters, the more importance registered medical practitioners are likely to have in state affairs. The GMC is, as we shall see (Chapter 7), an elite body, including a number of titled persons (see Table 2.1).

However, the coming of the European Community (EC) has already curtailed the sovereignty which the GMC formerly exercised over biomedical practice in the UK. The GMC can and does control the freedom of medical practitioners who qualified 'overseas' in medical schools which it does not recognize. As we shall see in Chapter 9, such practitioners are subjected to tests of linguistic and clinical ability before they are permitted to practise

Table 2.1 The elite character of the GMC

	1976	1979	1984	1989
Lords		1		
Baronets	1			
Knights	6	6	4	4
Baronesses	1			
Dames			1	
Professors[a]	12	29	29	29
Reverends		1	1	
Total Council	46	94	94	102

[a] Of whom two are also knights in 1976 and 1979, and one in 1984 and 1989.

in the UK. 'Overseas' in this context means anywhere outside the EC. The Treaty of Rome gives any doctor who is a properly qualified EC national the automatic right to register and practise in the UK. A potential employing authority may request a linguistic test before employing such a doctor, but the GMC cannot do so. The Council has no jurisdiction over medical education in member states of the EC. Its sovereignty is confined to those qualified in the UK and those seeking to enter the country from outside the EC. However, once registered in the UK, an EC-qualified EC national is subject to the same controls as other registered medical practitioners.

Other bodies, of course, play their part in the regulation of the profession. Much is done by the royal colleges, the universities and other medical societies, including the BMA, to maintain and enhance knowledge and practice. The Department of Health, formerly the Department of Health and Social Security (DHSS), the Welsh Office, the Scottish Home and Health Department, the health authorities and the Health Service Commissioner have responsibilities with regard to health care provided within the National Health Service (NHS). The role of the Council as the statutory body regulating the profession is, however, unique. Patients in private practice have no recourse except to the law courts or to the GMC.

I mentioned earlier that the BMA is often popularly confused with the GMC. However, these two bodies are quite distinct. The GMC, as we have seen, is a statutory body charged by Act of Parliament with responsibility for regulating the profession in such a manner that the public may know to whom they may reliably turn for medical advice; the BMA is a voluntary association of medical practitioners concerned to improve what in industrial relations terms would be called their terms and conditions of service. To this end the BMA is anxious to ensure that its members offer high and reliable standards of health care. The BMA seeks to influence the GMC on behalf of its members and in matters it sees as being in the interests of medicine in general. At the same time the GMC is, or at least some of its members are, sometimes frustrated by limitations upon its powers imposed by the BMA (and also by other bodies) through pressure in the parliamentary process.

However, neither the BMA nor any of the other bodies involved, powerful though some of them undoubtedly are (I think particularly of the royal colleges), can determine what undergraduate education shall be recognized for admission to the register nor can they remove the right to practise.

3
Historical Background: 1856–1968[1]

The birth of clinical medicine

There a general consensus that modern clinical medicine arose around the turn of the nineteenth century, emerging from eighteenth century beginnings in hospitals and clinics in France, Italy, Scotland and, somewhat later, England. In England its emergence was associated with the re-establishment of the hospitals, most of which had been closed along with the monasteries by Henry VIII. The GMC itself was not established until mid-century.

Before the eighteenth century, and indeed persisting into the nineteenth, the greatest part of healing had been undertaken by women in the domestic domain. Women cared for others in childbirth, and knew how to make potions and lotions to relieve suffering. Only the aristocracy were served by qualified physicians, but aristocrats also had recourse to wise women. Some have left records testifying to the beneficient effects of the treatment these women gave them.

The qualifications physicians gained were those needed for a gentleman and rested heavily on theory rather than on bedside treatment. Originally much more like artisans or tradesmen, by the eighteenth century the skills and knowledge of the barber-surgeons were developing a great deal faster than those of the physicians. The third group of healers, the apothecaries, were organized in corporations as were the physicians and the barber-surgeons. The apothecaries were only supposed to dispense, but in fact diagnosed as well despite the physicians attempts to control them; indeed this became legal in 1815.

In addition to these three formally organized groups, composed exclusively of men, and the women healers working in their own homes and helping others in the domestic domain, there was a wide variety of itinerant healers, bone setters, teeth pullers and others. Some of them were simply charlatans, but exploitation of gullible and suffering folk was not the exclusive province of those whom the rising professionals described as quacks; some of the rising professionals behaved in much the same way themselves.

Out of this miscellaneous array of healing modes allopathy, which was to become present-day biomedicine, emerged and became established as the dominant mode. Within 200 years the clinical successors of the allopathic healers had come to dominate over all others in Europe and North America and gained a pervasive influence throughout the world. The event is somewhat remarkable because at the outset the skills of allopathy had not been demonstrated as a more powerful healing mode.

Changes in the division of health labour

Many historical accounts of the development of our contemporary division of health labour are dominated by accounts of the tripartite division between physicians, surgeons and apothcaries which pertained until the nineteenth century, and of the struggles among them about rights to practise and the type of practice permitted. However, the divisions in practice were probably never so clear cut as the received wisdom has suggested. In the new hospitals the division between physicians and surgeons began to be replaced during the early nineteenth century by one between hospital doctors and those practising entirely from their own homes outside the hospital. That latter group, using skills of physicians, surgeons and apothecaries, later came to be known as general practitioners. But it was in association with the hospitals that the new clinical medicine was taught and here the medical schools developed.

A time of great change, the nineteenth century was also one of great competition among medical practitioners, as it was among manufacturers and traders. Practitioners of allopathic medicine who had undertaken relatively lengthy and expensive training, receiving qualifications from universities or from one or more of the medical corporations (physicians, surgeons or apothecaries), resented the competition from those not formally qualified, and felt cheated out of a just return on their educational investment. Practitioners felt the profession to be overcrowded. It seems there was an over provision in the 1830s and 1840s—in terms, that is, of what the population could afford. State-supported registration of the qualified was seen as an answer to this problem. General practitioners in particular felt that unqualified practice should be rendered illegal; those who worked among the poorer sections of the population felt the competition from the unqualified most keenly. This is one example of the many ways in which the material, as well as the practical day-to-day, interests of the hospital consultants, both physicians and surgeons, converged but diverged from those of general practitioners.

Establishing the new regulatory body

In these changed circumstances the established methods of medical regulation no longer fitted the conditions of practice. The long-standing and powerful control exerted by the medical corporations was felt to be particularly inappropriate. These resentments added fuel to the fire of the movement for reform. From the time the first Medical Reform Bill was introduced in 1840, until 1858 when the successful bill was introduced by W. F. Cowper, many bills had been laid before the House. The delay was caused by the divided interests among the practitioners and the associated failure to gain government support. Although the 1858 Act which established the General Council of Medical Education and Registration (the name was not shortened to the General Medical Council until 1951) flowed from Cowper's Bill, it was much different from his initial proposals.

Cowper's Bill intended that the term 'qualified medical practitioner' should imply that the practitioner was not only legally entitled to practise but also was well-qualified. Entry qualifications should reflect competence in all the major branches of practice, medicine, surgery and midwifery. This proposal was in line with what general practitioners wanted, but was in direct opposition to all the colleges, who wanted to keep their several qualifications distinct. The colleges won this one: the provision that all registered practitioners should be qualified in all major branches of medicine was lost.

As to the composition of the Council, the bill proposed the medical corporations should be represented, as should the universities; there were also to be six independent members nominated by the Crown. This gave a possibility, but no assurance, that there might be general practitioner members. Lobbying by the colleges ensured that this part of the bill was amended in their favour. A proviso that the six nominated members should not include members of any of the corporations was also lost, being replaced by a requirement that there should be four from England and one each from Scotland and Ireland. The General Council of Medical Education and Registration as finally enacted was composed of representatives of all the nineteen separate licensing bodies. There were 24 members in all: nine members represented the royal colleges; seven represented the four English and three Irish universities; two represented the four Scottish universities; and six were nominated by the Queen on the advice of the Privy Council. General practitioners had no places. Thus the formerly established medical leadership remained in control. The royal colleges had avoided, for the time being at least, the curtailment of their powers which the wide-ranging authority that was originally proposed would have imposed.

The powers of the Council were

> slender and vaguely expressed ... and it was hard for it to assert its authority which was opposed by those well established institutions that were represented upon it ... The opposition was especially difficult as it was both without and within the Council.
>
> Richardson (1983), p. 8

In terms of standardizing medical education the Council at first stressed the importance of education 'to be men' and, from 1861, required that candidates should have passed an examination in the arts to a standard approved by the Council (Bhattacharya, 1983, p. 19). Four years of professional studies were to follow an examination in general education. Nearly ten years after its foundation the Council in 1867 agreed on ten medical subjects (descriptive and general anatomy, physiology, chemistry, material medica, practical pharmacy, medicine, surgery, midwifery, forensic medicine) which should be obligatory in terms of teaching and examination. But the Council still did not have powers to forbid registration to those who lacked such an all-round medical education.

Establishing the profession: the advantages of the single register

The general practitioners had been in favour of the provision that all practitioners should be listed alphabetically in a single register. This raised 'for the College of Physicians the awful prospect that in law the activities of the physician might be seen in the same light as those of a common tradesman' (Waddington, 1984, p. 110). The provision of the single register within which all were equal under the simple definition of 'registered medical practitioner' proved of immense importance in creating and maintaining the unity of the profession. It represented a move away from purely local arrangements for regulation to a more centralized system. Furthermore, in establishing the single register the Act stressed what all practitioners had in common rather than those characteristics which divided them.

Ultimately, weak though the original Council was, the 1858 Act proved crucial for the establishment of medicine as a profession. It led to the development of a self-conscious occupation aiming for control of work situation and client, controlling its own labour supply and its own remuneration. The Act did not ban practitioners of kinds other than those the Council were prepared to register, nor have they been banned since. What such persons were, and still are, not permitted to do is to advertise themselves as 'registered medical practitioners'. General practitioners probably had more to gain from registration than the hospital consultants, for, as had been noted, they experienced more competition from those unqualified in allopathy, including the women healers, than did the consultants.

Registration and the definition of the 'registered medical practitioner' may not have created a formal monopoly of practice for the allopathists, but it did create a monopoly for the registered in all public institutions and government medical services. This was to become increasingly important as the years went by. Unregistered practitioners could not, from the time the register was established, certify any statutory documents. They were excluded from the medical list, 'the panel', under the 1911 Health Insurance Act. The coming of the NHS in 1948 further restricted the field of their activities. The unregistered who wish to work autonomously are forced to practise privately. Resources for research and practice have not flowed to them or their organizations on the scale which registered medical practitioners and their organizations have enjoyed. However, historically in Britain unregistered practitioners have been free to practise, a situation now threatened by the European Community.

Controlling the supply of labour

As was later made plain to the 1882 Royal Commission on the Medical Acts, another effect of establishing the Council was a reduction in the level of recruitment to the profession, presumably a result of raising the entry requirements. In the 1860s and 1870s the growth in the number of registered medical practitioners was minimal, less proportionately than the growth in the size of the general population. The restriction of entry to the more highly qualified had a further consequence of raising the status and remuneration of the registered practitioners. Complaints of overcrowding ceased. Indeed, by the late 1870s and 1880s a shortage of practitioners was generally recognized.

The excessive competition which came from 'overcrowding' was also associated with complaints of ungentlemanly or unprofessional conduct as between one practitioner and another. In part these disputes were connected with the new division of labour which was being established among practitioners. For example, many general practitioners complained that consultants poached their patients. Once set up, the Council was in a position to establish standards of intra-professional conduct backed up by disciplinary procedures, and thus to begin to develop a national system of medical ethics.

Medical impetus for registration

Looking back on the establishment of the Council in 1858 it seems clear that the impetus came from medicine—it was a desire to create circumstances in which their income and status could be improved that led medical men to press for reform of medical regulation. Whatever their differences, all were agreed on the importance of regulation for the help it would be to them in controlling who could practise, thereby reducing competition. Contrary to the beliefs of many, the interests of the public were a secondary, not a primary, consideration.

These two aspects of protection and privilege were stressed in the GMC's evidence to the Merrison Committee at a time when the Council was under considerable attack and were made generally available in the 1974 pamphlet 'Constitution and Functions'. Although stating that it laid upon the Council a general duty to protect the public, the evidence pointed out that the 1858 Act

> was passed largely as a result of initiative within the profession, and the establishment of the Council was desired as much for the protection of the duly qualified medical practitioner from the competition of unqualified practitioners as for the protection of the public. Registration confers a number of privileges. For example, only registered practitioners may hold medical appointments in the National Health Service or in the public services or Armed Forces, prescribe or supply dangerous or other restricted drugs, give statutory certificates and recover at law fees for medical advice and attendance. Fully registered practitioners may also claim exemption from jury service.
>
> GMC Minutes, CX (1973), p. 179

The establishment of the Council ensured the triumph of allopathy and made possible the profession of medicine as it is today.

Consolidating the profession

The 1886 Act further consolidated the profession. It provided that the profession as a whole should elect representatives to the Council (although only five out of a total of 30 members), thus removing a major source of general practitioners' discontent. However, the Council itself was given power to increase the number of the elected if it so wished. The presence of elected members may have been mainly of symbolic importance, but it was a further move in the direction of a united profession under the General Council.

A second important change was the 1886 requirement that entry qualifications for the register had from now on to include proficiency in medicine, surgery and midwifery. This clearly increased the power of the Council over against the medical corporations in so far as what we now call basic medical education is concerned. It increased the commonality among all registered practitioners, thereby further enhancing unity of the profession. The inclusion of both medicine and surgery in the basic qualifications can be seen as the final dissolution, in legal terms at least, of the former major distinction between medicine and surgery. The inclusion of midwifery has to be seen in rather a different light.

The triumph of obstetrics over midwifery

Since the eighteenth century medical doctors had increasingly been practising midwifery, a previously all-woman occupation, probably felt to be polluting for men. The very name, man-midwives, by which medical men who assisted at births were originally known, indicates the ambiguity of their status. Also known in the early period as accoucheurs, they later settled for the term obstetrician. Delivering the children of the rising middle classes was an important way in which general practitioners increased their clientele.

Opposition to the new practice of obstetrics came from medical men who thought that midwifery was not an appropriate activity for a man, especially a gentleman and a doctor. It came also from women midwives, who are unlikely to have been as incompetent as the medical men made out. As in the case with the campaigns against the unqualified, historical reality and propaganda have become confused. Most likely in this, as in all branches of the healing arts, the competent and the incompetent could be found. The inclusion of midwifery as a necessary essential qualification for all registered medical practitioners in the 1886 Act marked a triumph for the new over the conservative medical practice and for the male doctors over the women midwives.

A man's profession

The General Council, composed as it was of members of the royal colleges and the medical schools, was also composed entirely of men. This male preserve was immediately challenged by Elizabeth Blackwell who had, not without difficulty, been permitted to qualify as a medical practitioner in America. She was able to demonstrate that she had been practising medicine in England before the medical register was established under the 1858 Act. The medical gentlemen had no choice but to admit her. However, they quickly blocked that entry route by barring foreign qualifications for the future. When Elizabeth Garrett slipped through a loophole by getting private tuition and taking the apothecaries' examination, the General Council made sure that that route was blocked too.

The story of the determined attempt to keep women out of medicine has been told many times, as has the women's at least as determined efforts to be permitted to qualify and practise. This is not the place go into the detail of that struggle. It is, however, worth noting that in 1875, in response to the Privy Council, which was seeking opinions on a bill to permit the recognition of foreign degrees held by women, the General Council of Medical Education concluded:

> The Council are of the opinion that the study and practice of medicine and surgery instead of affording a field of exertion well fitted for women, present special difficulties which cannot safely be ignored ... but the Council are not prepared to say that women ought to be excluded.
>
> Quoted in Scott (1984), p. 1766

The overriding consideration seems to have been that the universities' freedom should not be interfered with by legislation. If women were admitted, their education and examination should be conducted entirely apart from men.

Women on the Council

Table 3.1 shows the increase in the total number of registered medical practitioners from 1858 to 1971. The slow but inexorable increase in the numbers of women doctors after those early struggles can be seen but no medical woman was elected to the Council until 1933, 75 years after its formation. Sadly Dr Christine Murrell died before she could take her seat. A medical woman was nominated by the Privy Council in 1950–1955 and

Table 3.1 The increasing number of women doctors and their representation on the GMC

Year	Number on register	Number on Council
1871	2	0
1881	25	0
1891	100	0
1901	200	0
1911	600	0
1921	1 500	0
1931	3 300	0
1951	7 520	1
1971	12 596	1

Sources: Scott (1984), p. 1766; Pyke-Lees (1958); *GMC Annual Report for 1976*.

one, but only one, was elected from 1955 until 1979. Since then there have been a few more women on the Council (see Chapter 7).

A lay council or a lay voice?

Before 1858 one proposal had been that a body of lay men should regulate the profession—a far cry from the Council composed entirely of medical men that eventually emerged. Not until the 1950 Medical Act was statutory provision made for lay members on the Council. That Act provided for eight Crown nominees of whom three should be lay. However, from 1926 the king had included one lay person among those whom he nominated. Bernard Shaw is said to have claimed credit for this, believing that the public should maintain vigilance over the Council, especially in matters of discipline. In 1950 and again from 1955 onwards the lay Crown nominees included a woman.

By the time the Second World War broke out, the Council had increased in size to 42: 38 medical members, of whom seven were now elected (the number had been increased in 1909 and 1931 by Order in Council); one lay member; and three dentists. As well as providing for lay members the 1950 Medical Act (which followed the Goodenough Report of 1944) increased the total size of the Council to 50, providing for: 44 medical members (11 elected; five Crown nominees; 28 appointed by universities and royal colleges etc.); three lay members; and three dentists. (The 1957 Act which set up the General Dental Council finally ended the GMC's direct responsibility for dental surgeons.)

The pre-registration year, inspection and discipline

The 1950 Act also made three other important changes. First, from 1953 every doctor who had qualified was to spend a period as a resident house officer in an approved hospital before being fully registered. The details were left to the Council, which nominated a year, to be known as the pre-registration year, six months of which were to be spent in medicine and six months in surgery, except that up to six months could be spent in mid-wifery or up to six months in a health centre in place of either medicine or surgery. The consolidating Act of 1956 made the pre-registration year the responsibility of the universities. Second, while before the 1950 Act the Council had the right to visit or inspect examinations of universities and licensing authorities, this was now extended to the visitation of teaching in medical schools. Third, apparently not welcomed by the Council, the Act established the disciplinary committee; previously the entire Council had sat on disciplinary cases.

In response the Council determined that cases of conduct, i.e. an allegation of infamous professional conduct, should be heard by all 19 members of the disciplinary committee, while cases of conviction in the courts should be heard by panels of nine members of that committee. Furthermore the whole Council would now become responsible for education rather than a standing committee as heretofore.

Shedding the pharmacopoeia

When the General Council was established in 1858, it had been given responsibility for publishing a *British Pharmacopoeia*. In the mid-twentieth century it discharged this function through a Pharmacopoeia Committee which met twice yearly, receiving reports from the British Pharmacopoeia Commission. This responsibility was transferred to the Department of Health and Social Security in 1968.

The power of the presidents

In the early part of the twentieth century probably there was less turbulence around or in the Council than in either the earlier or the later periods. This was perhaps particularly true during the long period of office of Sir David Campbell who, according to the then registrar, took a somewhat passive view of the Council's role so far as education, discipline and overseas registration was concerned. The way in which the Council was constituted at the outset left a good deal of space for action under Orders to be made by the Privy Council as well as rules and regulations to be made by the General Council itself, a tradition which has continued.

The Acts have also given a good deal of power to the office of president. The names of the presidents, their terms of office and their ages when their term finished are shown in Table 3.2. The president's stance has greatly affected the work of the Council. Lord Cohen, who took office in 1961, was more active in a number of respects than his predecessor. The disciplinary activity of the Council increased markedly. The number of days the committee sat per year increased from an average of six from 1955 to 1961 to over 16 from 1962 to 1973 (*GMC Minutes, CXI*, 1974, xix–xx). During Lord Cohen's term of office the disturbances described in the next chapter started. There were many reasons for these—it would not be appropriate to lay the responsibility for them at Lord Cohen's door. He was, however, an important actor in how they were handled.

Table 3.2 Terms of office of presidents of the GMC

Period	President	Time in office in years	Age on completion of term of office
1858–60	Sir Benjamin Brodie	$1\frac{1}{2}$	77
1860–63	Mr Green	$3\frac{1}{2}$	72
1864–69	Sir George Burrows	$5\frac{1}{2}$	69
1868–74	Sir George Paget	5	63
1874–87	Sir Henry Acland	$12\frac{3}{4}$	72
1887–91	Mr Marshall	$3\frac{1}{2}$	73
1891–98	Sir Richard Quain	$6\frac{3}{4}$	81
1898–1904	Sir William Turner	$6\frac{1}{2}$	73
1904–31	Sir Donald MacAlister	27	77
1931–39	Sir Norman Walker	8	77
1939–49	Sir Herbert Eason	10	75
1949–61	Sir David Campbell	12	73
1961–73	Lord Cohen of Birkenhead	12	73
1973–80	Sir John (now Lord) Richardson	$6\frac{1}{2}$	70
1980–81	Sir Robert Wright	$1\frac{1}{2}$	66
1982–89	Sir John (now Lord) Walton	7	67
1989–	Sir Robert Kilpatrick		

Sources: *GMC Minutes, CXVII* (1980), p. 54; *GMC Annual Report for 1981*, p. 2; *GMC Annual Report for 1982*, p. 2.

The Council in 1968

By 1968, 110 years after the Council was first enacted, the GMC was an established body, central to the UK medical profession, now an occupation of high status and prestige and well reputed world-wide. Despite the reforms, the GMC still bore many of the marks of its origin, both in terms of the high aspirations of its founders and of the rivalries and jealousies in the many branches of medicine. The Council was by now responsible for a profession whose skills, and the tools available to it, had increased immeasurably since its foundation—skills and tools which had immense power to heal and to harm if misused. As the Merrison Committee (1975) later put it, when the Council was established by Act of Parliament, the profession had entered into a contract with the state whereby medical practitioners were granted the privilege of professional self-regulation in exchange for ensuring that the public were able to trust the competence of those qualified practitioners whom they consulted. The task by 1968 was a great deal more onerous than it had been in 1858; the number of practitioners to be regulated had increased vastly. There had also been qualitative changes in the nature of medicine and its complexity.

Note

1.   Sources used in this chapter include: Arney (1982), Bhattacharya (1983), Bynum and Porter (1987), Clark (1968), Donnison (1988), Draper (1983), *GMC Minutes*, CX (1973), Apps III and VII, Loudon (1986), Oakley (1976), Pelling (1987), Peterson (1978), Porter (1982, 1987), Pyke-Lees (1958), Richardson (1983), Scott (1984, 1986), Stacey (1988a), Waddington (1984), Walton (1979), Wood (1987).

PART 2

THE DECADE OF THE PROFESSION

4

The Professional Revolt

The 1960s were iconoclastic years, with the Beatles, the mini-skirt, the world-wide student uprising of 1968—social, cultural and political change was in the air. The consequences were still working through in the mid-1970s. Medicine did not escape these movements. For the GMC they marked the beginning of the end of the tranquil years.

The NHS was included in government preoccupation with administrative reorganization. Kenneth Robinson, Secretary of State for Health and Social Services, introduced the first green paper to propose the integration of the three branches of the NHS (hospital, family practitioner and local authority) in 1968. This was followed, when the government changed, by Richard Crossman's 1970 green paper, hard on the heels of which came Keith Joseph's 1971 consultative document when the government changed yet again. The planning and implementation of this first major health service reorganization, finally enacted in 1974, raised a great many anxieties among everyone connected with the NHS.

The medical profession also wrestled during these years with continuing problems about medical pay and its comparability with earnings abroad. What's more, there was also the 1968 Todd Report on medical education with, among many other recommendations, its suggestion of specialist registers. This threatened the authority of the royal colleges and raised fears among rank and file general practitioners, that they might once again be put into some kind of second-class medical category.

Such was the background to the professional revolt, focused on the GMC, which came to a head in 1970–1972. The revolutionary fire was fuelled by discontent with many aspects of medical professional structure and organization. There was the historical discontent of the GPs, whose initial unhappiness with the GMC had never really been satisfied. The College of General Practitioners, founded in 1952, became a royal college in December 1967, but still had no seat on the Council. In establishing the College and then seeking through training to make a specialism out of their very generalism, the GPs had made a bid to join the medical hierarchy, albeit in a more modern and democratic version of the long-established college mode of professional organisation.

Opposition to the medical establishment

Much of the discontent was with the nature of the medical establishment. There was discontent at the most senior level. Regional consultants felt they were excluded from a proper place in the NHS and in the colleges, that their interests were not properly represented. As one put it: 'the elite of St Thomas's, Westminster, St Bartholomew's and St Mary's had control of the negotiating procedure and the whole profession'. This was an arrangement which antedated the NHS. Consultants were no longer concentrated, as they had previously been, in London but were scattered all over the country in NHS hospitals. Regional consultants with other specialists consequently formed a separate organization, the Hospital Consultants and Specialists Association, to press for their interests. In their view GPs were better represented in seats of power than they were.

There was also a great deal of discontent among junior hospital doctors (i.e. all those hospital doctors who did not have consultant status) about their pay, conditions of work and the attitudes of their seniors towards them. Some were discontented with the Hospital Junior Staffs Group Council of the BMA. They felt there was no forum in which their points of view were properly expressed and listened to, let alone acted on. They organized into the Junior Hospital Doctors Association (JHDA) which published a journal *On Call*. Underlying the JHDA's discontent was the hierarchical nature of medical organization in medical schools, hospitals and professional organizations. The JHDA shared with other hospital doctors concern about the hospital staffing structure, specifically what should be the proportion of consultants to other grades. Furthermore, the JHDA, and also other groups of doctors, included the leadership of the BMA in their anti-establishment feelings. These organizations and many rank and file members in the late 1960s and early 1970s increasingly believed that the BMA leadership did not have rank and file interests at heart, but instead was effectively part of the medical establishment.

With regard to the GMC itself, rank and file practitioners resented the fact that elected members were in a minority on the Council. Junior hospital doctors, none of whom were on the GMC, now joined GPs in this. For junior hospital doctors, being by definition in the senior ranks neither of the universities nor the royal colleges, election was the only likely route to a seat.

The GMC's problems

The General Medical Council had its own problems. These included the retention fee, the control of 'sick doctors', the regulation of overseas doctors, the improper prescribing of drugs of addiction and the proposals for a specialist register.

As early as 1963 the Council had identified a severe financial problem, derived from three sources: the increased work it had to do consequent upon the very success of biomedicine and the increased numbers of doctors practising or seeking to practise; its own diligence in undertaking more work; and, finally, inflation. The only resolution the Council could see was to require an annual retention fee from all registered medical practitioners. As things stood doctors paid an initial fee when they were admitted to the register which then lasted them for life unless they were removed for some reason and had to re-register i.e. apply for restoration to the register. To require an annual fee was thus a new departure and one which would require legislation.

A second problem the Council had identified was how to handle doctors who were not fit to practise by reason of mental illness (often but not always alcohol or drug dependence). The powers of the Council offered no way to deal with such doctors except throuh the disciplinary procedures; the 'mad' could not be differentiated from the 'bad'. The Council could only impose penalties such as removal from the register or admonishment on these ill people—the first left no chance for recovery and rehabilitation, the second did not adequately protect the public. Any resolution of this problem would also require legislation.

A third difficulty had to do with the large number of doctors qualified overseas who had been and were being recruited to fill vacancies in the NHS. There was increasing anxiety within the profession, among nursing and other health workers and among the general public, about the linguistic and clinical skills of such doctors who, while it was agreed that the NHS relied utterly on their services, were coming to be seen as a 'problem'. In addition, their mode of registration (necessary before they could practise in the UK) constituted problems for the doctors themselves and for their employers (see Chapter 5).

While sometimes overlapping with the problem of drug-addicted doctors, the question of the misprescribing of dangerous drugs was a different one. In the 1960s some doctors were identified (Dr Peto's case was the most notorious) who were misusing their professional powers by prescribing drugs of addiction other than for the *bona fide* treatment of patients, i.e. for their own profit they were providing addicts with drugs. The illicit taking of drugs of dependence was increasingly being defined politically as a major social problem, so the behaviour of these doctors was seen as a particularly reprehensible abuse of professional privilege. The GMC undoubtedly could be said to have responsibilities in this regard.

The Todd Report also had implications for the GMC, notably its recommendations about undergraduate medical education. Furthermore, if there was to be specialist registration' should not the Council be responsible for it? And who but the Council might be responsible for the generality of continuing medical education? But these suggestions were not acceptable to the royal colleges, whose prerogative specialist training had always been; they were not likely to be supported by college representatives on the Council.

Council sought a medical act to cope with some of these problems, namely the control of overseas-qualified doctors and sick doctors, and also to give powers to levy an annual retention fee. It did nothing about tighter controls on the improper prescribing of drugs of addiction, nor did it seek powers to establish a specialist register.

Legislation

Finally, in May 1969 the Medical Bill which the Council wanted came before the House of Lords. It gave Council powers to levy an annual retention fee, proposed changes in the registration arrangements for overseas doctors, and, as an addition to the sole punishment of erasure, proposed powers to suspend doctors' registrations for not more than 12 months, including power to suspend 'forthwith' if a case was sufficienty serious. This last was designed to provide more flexibility in handling 'sick doctors'.

Government took action on the issues the GMC had left out. It had already in 1967 moved the Dangerous Drugs Bill which included provision for a special tribunal to deal with malprescribing doctors. In July 1969 Richard Crossman, Secretary of State, gave notice of his intention to legislate for a register of specialists along the lines recommended by the Todd Report.

The first proposal became law with the establishment of the drug squad and special powers given to the Home Office to control malprescribing doctors. This left the GMC having simply to handle those who were convicted of prescribing drugs of addiction for other than *bona fide* reasons. Some doctors felt the GMC had been wrong to let this control go to government. As to the specialist register, Crossman received strong protests from the BMA that they were being given too little time to consider the idea, opposition from general practitioners and, apparently, although this was not made so public, strong opposition from the Royal College of Physicians. Crossman withdrew his proposal.

The 1969 Bill

The idea of suspension had been floated by members in the *British Medical Journal* (*BMJ*) for some years. Enough doctors recognized the limitations of there being only one way to remove a doctor from the register, so the BMA after much discussion ultimately recommended acceptance of this. It was the provision that was going to touch all doctors' pockets which created opposition to the GMC.

The proposed retention fee had been reported in the medical press in May 1966. The BMA and the *BMJ* at that time both supported the GMC, although the *BMJ* published a letter of protest from Francis Pigott, who later became one of the major campaigners for GMC reform. It seems Pigott was not alone in his objections. The 1966 Annual Representative Meeting (ARM), contrary to the BMA council's advice, carried a motion against the 'savage and quite unreasonable' GMC fee proposals. Subsequent discussions in the BMA council revealed divisions of opinion. While some members thought the annual fee should be paid, one member said that since the state wanted the profession regulated, it should pay—a suggestion often repeated in the following years. Later that year, in July, a motion put at ARM opposing the annual retention fee was lost, but another, that the level of the proposed fee (at £2) was too high, was carried. Already in 1965 the ARM had passed a resolution calling for better representation of GPs on the GMC. In the 1966 debate the question of the proportion of elected members on the GMC was raised again.

Despite the rank and file opposition to the retention fee, Dr Ronald Gibson, the chairperson, insisted the BMA could not withdraw its support for the GMC's proposals. An important argument was the loss of professional independence which government funding of the GMC would involve. So hostile was the profession to the GMC that ARM debated a motion to abolish the GMC and replace it by the BMA's own council, on the grounds that the latter was a democratic body. That motion was defeated, but another, that elected members should be in a majority on the GMC, was carried and the cry of 'no taxation without representation' was raised.

Resistance to the fee

The legislation empowering the GMC to charge an annual retention fee received the royal assent on 25 July 1969. From 1970 doctors would have to pay if they wished to remain registered. One might have expected a good bit of whingeing and then for the whole affair to fade out, especially as the charge was small compared with what doctors were accustomed to pay for their professional organization memberships and, furthermore, they could reclaim the fees as practice expenses or tax deductible, depending on their employment circumstances. Resistance did not subside; indeed it was enhanced in 1970 and thereafter.

The iconoclasm—disputes not contained

Differences and divisions within the medical profession are by no means uncommon: in face of this, its continued unity since the mid-nineteenth century has in many ways been quite remarkable. The unusual feature of the divisions and dissensions in the later part of the 1960s and the early 1970s was the profession's failure to contain these domestic difficulties within the walls of medical council chambers and common rooms: the row spilled into the national press and ultimately reached Parliament. This was the iconoclasm—the disputes got outside the 'club', indeed were taken there by defiant acts of some of the club members themselves.

Several thousand doctors refused to pay the annual retention fee and were threatened with erasure. If erased they would be unable to practise; without them the proper functioning of the NHS was threatened. This led to government intervention. How was it that this dispute was not contained?

Origins of the revolt

The many discontents in the profession which helped to fuel the rebellion had been around for a long time: it was the annual retention fee which provided the trigger for opposition to the GMC and thus a focus for the discontents. The lack of adequate rank and file representation in the medical establishment was seen as an explanation of its failure to handle the problems in the profession effectively.

Some senior members of the profession laid the origins of the revolt at the door of the BMA. Others said it all began 'in those little papers *Pulse* and *World Medicine*' ('little' here seems to refer more to how the establishment perceived the status of these papers than to their size). Some believed that Michael O'Donnell, then editor of *World Medicine*, could be held responsible, while others implied that *Pulse* had an equal share. Other observers blamed the intransigence of the GMC itself in not being prepared to propose an increase in the number of elected members at an early stage of the difficulties.

The role of the medical press[1]

The leadership's impression that the rebellion had its origin in the 'little papers' may have had much to do with the press's lack of interest in the

GMC before the late 1960s. The *BMJ* reported regularly, in great detail and with full names and circumstances, the cases heard before the disciplinary committee. So did *The Lancet*, but in a more summary manner, not always including charges but also giving names and outcomes. There were few articles discussing the GMC's role or functions. In 1965 the *BMJ* had a leader on the Privy Council's attitude to appeals from the disciplinary committee and a letter calling for power to suspend. *The Lancet* focussed on problems concerning overseas doctors. Neither overlooked the proposed annual retention fee, however.

From a situation in which the GMC was little noticed in the early 1960s, by the end of the decade, the Council had become the focus of a great deal of professional and journalistic attention, anxiety and hostility. However, nothing that had gone before could equal what was to come in 1970.

Pulse had given space to questions of overseas doctors' registration and to sick doctors in 1967, and in 1968 to GMC warnings about persons offering false qualifications and again to overseas doctors. However, in 1969 it began to show more than occasional interest in GMC-related issues. In that year overseas doctors, the annual retention fee (when the Bill was laid before Parliament), specialist registration, junior doctors and regional consultants, were featured, in that order of first mention. No letters were published from doctors in response to the news of the Bill, which contained powers for an annual retention fee.

World Medicine enters

In contrast to the *BMJ*, *The Lancet* and *Pulse*, *World Medicine* made no comment until 28 August 1969, a full month after the Act had received the royal assent. Fresh to the fray, Michael O'Donnell headed a page 1 'News Item' 'Why should we pay to stay on register, ask angry doctors'. A leader (Michael O'Donnell was the editor) suggested the GMC was far too expensive. Furthermore, using the analogy of the judiciary, the editor described as 'ridiculous' the suggestion that if the government supported the GMC the medical profession would lose its independence. The attack was as much against the BMA leadership for letting the situation arise as it was against the GMC. Regretting that ARM had not supported opposition to the annual levy, the editor thought doctors should make their views about it known 'before the damage is done'.

He followed this in September by including a reply-paid postcard asking for readers' opinions. The notice about this was printed alongside a 'News In Brief' article drawing attention to JHDA opposition to paying the retention fee and suggesting that any protest would have to be well organized. Michael O'Donnell pointed out that although the GMC now had power to charge an annual retention fee it was not compelled to do so. A week after the survey was launched he was asking 'Do we need the GMC?', a theme he returned to in December.

Rebellion spreads

By 13 January 1970 the postal survey showed 11,540 doctors were against the levy and only 466 in favour. As *Pulse* put it, 'Suddenly—as though overnight—the respect previously accorded [the GMC] by the rank-and-file of the profession has dramatically diminished, and many doctors are now not only critical of its working but openly alarmed by its apparent climb to totalitarian power' (31 January 1970, p. 7).

In November the GMC had confirmed the retention fee would be £2—the original intention to charge £3 had been reduced to £2 in negotiations with the BMA. Coincidentally the BMA was to raise its subscription in 1970, a move which critics did not fail to point out. In February *World Medicine* was calling for a thorough reorganization of the BMA.

As 1970 progressed, doctors who had no intention of paying the annual fee made their feelings known, some diffusely raising many complaints, but more linking their objections to the precise demand 'no taxation without representation'. *World Medicine* encouraged BMA branches to become active in the campaign. The BMA council was charged by members who supported that demand with having acted illegally in agreeing an annual retention fee with the GMC in opposition to a resolution passed at the 1969 ARM in Aberdeen of the Representative Body (RB: BMA members meeting in the Annual Representative Meetings—ARMs—or in Special Representative Meetings—SRMs—constitute the RB of the Association). Legal opinion supported the rebels (BMA council, 7 January 1970): the RB and not council had power to speak for the BMA. So the BMA council asked the GMC and the Privy Council to delay action on the annual retention fee until an SRM already called for May. However, Lord Cohen (GMC president) reportedly refused to ask the Privy Council for a postponement beyond 12 February. Consequently an SRM was called for 12 February. *World Medicine* continued its agitation against the 'levy' in preparation for this meeting, as did *Pulse*.

SRM demands conditions before payment

The SRM was long and complex; the *BMJ Supplement* report (21 February 1970) took a full 12 pages. SRM agreed to the BMA council's recommendation to accept the £2 annual fee only on conditions namely: a majority of elected members on the GMC, adequate places for elected members on GMC committees, and an immediate review of the functions and composition of the GMC, these to be agreed between the RB (specifically), the GMC and the government. If an annual retention fee were to be imposed against the profession's wishes, the BMA should advise members of the medical profession to withhold payment of fees. A reported last-minute message from Lord Cohen that the GMC would agree to a majority of elected members cut no ice. The BMA council at once met in emergency session. It proposed that a single £2 fee should be paid for that year, but that the principle of an annual retention fee should not be accepted until the SRM conditions, just voted on, were fulfilled. This was agreed and doctors were consequently advised *not* to withhold fees for the time being. Despite their militant mood, SRM were finding it difficult to 'go the whole hog'.

The *Lancet*, although agreeing that the GMC's functions could do with review, thought it had been 'a black day' for the BMA and the profession. In The *Lancet's* eyes 'the possibility of BMA control [of the GMC was] too substantial a spectre to be ignored' (21 February 1970, pp. 396–397). The BMA, it argued, is devoted to protecting professional interests while the duty of the GMC is to protect the public. The *BMJ* (21 February 1970), on the other hand, urged doctors to pay the single retention fee for 1970 to gain time for negotiations in which the BMA should take the lead. The leader writer was anxious that if any large number of doctors refused to pay and were consequently erased from the register, government would be faced with a disruption of the NHS. It might then not only pay for the regulation of the profession, but take it over. 'The dangers of this to a profession already employed by the State in a National Health Service are too obvious to need stressing' (*BMJ*, 21 February 1970, p. 446). In contrast *Pulse* asked 'Do we really need the GMC?' (21 February 1970, p. 6), suggesting the Department of Health could just as well keep the register.

The CMO intervenes

Government was indeed alarmed by SRM's action. On 11 March the Chief Medical Officer (CMO) of England called the parties together. This meeting led ultimately to the establishment of a joint working party with three representatives each of the universities, the royal colleges, and the BMA, with Sir Brynmor Jones, a lay member of the GMC, in the chair.[2]

Annual fees ordered

A fresh round of criticism was released when the Privy Council having, at the end of March, made an order to impose the retention fee, the GMC sent out notices informing practitioners the £2 fee was payable (including a banker's order form, implying the continuity the BMA had rejected) and saying that refusal to pay might, after due warning, lead to erasure from the register. Furthermore, as the *BMJ* first leader said, the joint working party had not yet come into existence; nevertheless it did not want the GMC to founder. *Pulse* was much more hostile, criticizing many aspects of the GMC's work and fully reporting the rebellious actions of the Liverpool and Merseyside BMA branch.

At the May SRM of the BMA, the Todd recommendations and the green paper on NHS reorganization featured at least as prominently as the retention fee issue. The JHDA-inspired motions urging BMA support for non-payers failed to gain majorities, the SRM agreeing to wait for the findings of the BMA/GMC working party. One aim of this, according to Dr Ronald Gibson, BMA council chairperson, was to keep the whole thing 'within the family'.

At the June 1970 meeting of the full GMC, Lord Cohen, as its president, made an extended statement answering the major criticisms to which the GMC had been subjected. At that meeting the GMC formally agreed to join in the working party on its structure. It did not, however, change its position about collecting the retention fees, which it saw as essential to solve its financial difficulties.

Defiant non-payers

In November non-payers received warning letters from the GMC. In December *Pulse* (5 December 1970) carried on its front page an open letter to the GMC from Francis Pigott explaining that he would not pay his retention fee, despite a final reminder, 'because I believe that the basic argument for the exclusive financing of the General Medical Council by the medical profession is of dubious morality, and the present constitution of the Council is unsatisfactory for the certain protection of the public interest'. He argued that the present constitution of the Council gave an in-built bias in favour of the medical profession; a large increase of non-medical members was needed and half the finance should come from government. The colleges and the BMA, not the GMC, existed to protect the profession. In Dr Pigott's view the time had come to review the functions, structure and financing of the GMC in the light of modern conditions—a review which should be undertaken by an independent public body.

GMC elections

Frances Pigott had been one among a number of candidates in a GMC by-election in 1970 occasioned by the death of a member. In the event John Fry, a prominent member of the Royal College of General Practitioners (RGCP), was elected. In 1971 the term of office of all 11 elected members would expire and elections be held. The BMA had warned members of this as early as March 1970. According to BMA custom the secretariat called for nominations for candidates whom the BMA would sponsor. ARM in July spent time selecting candidates—only to decide the next day to cease sponsorship. Given the negotiations over the GMC, the BMA felt it should keep its distance. Nevertheless an unprecedentedly large number of candidates stood for the 11 vacant seats.

Rebels elected

When the results, delayed by a postal strike, were declared John Fry, re-elected after a year's service, topped the poll—evidence of support for and from the RCGP. Apart from him, all those elected were new to the GMC. They included four who had been vociferous agitators for GMC reform, if not abolition: Kate Bradley, President of the JHDA, although technically no longer a junior since she had now obtained a consultant post; Francis Pigott, also a JHDA candidate; Myre Sim, who had been selected as a BMA candidate before that body withdrew sponsorship for 1971; and Michael O'Donnell. The last had put himself up despite having claimed in a *World Medicine* in December, 1969: 'Our job as journalists is to watch what is happening, to comment on what we see, but not become involved in the happenings themselves' (30 December 1969, p. 13). Generous to a rival editor, although not doing full justice to its own earlier publications, *Pulse* reported (8 May 1970, p. 1) 'if it was anyone's election, this was Michael O'Donnell's, for the issues were the ones to which he first drew attention in *World Medicine* and continued to press with a relentlessness which drew strictures in Presidential addresses'. The four referred to as 'young turks' were a disparate bunch, as Michael O'Donnell was to confirm to me 20 years later, differing on many issues, including the GMC. All they shared was opposition to the way the medical establishment was doing things.

Pulse (8 May 1970) described the election results as 'at least a partial victory for the militant element of the profession who have long campaigned for reforms', but only a partial victory because others elected were establishment figures, in which cateogory *Pulse* included John Fry and Frances Gardiner, the successful Medical Women's Federation (MWF) candidate. Furthermore, the 'establishment' was well entrenched in the university, college and society seats. The intention of the dissidents had been to use the fee issue to rock the establishment. Now these four found themselves sitting among its members and supporters. However, the election of the dissidents was by no means the last that was to be heard of the revolt.

Between the candidates putting up and the election results being declared, the Brynmor Jones working party had reported. This was the first of a series of enquiries into the GMC. The last was the official Merrison enquiry. How that public investigation came about and what it concluded is the subject of the next section.

The Brynmor Jones working party

The terms of reference of the working party concerned the composition of the Council. Questions of function which the BMA, the JDHA and others had wanted reviewed were not included. The report in March 1971 recommended an increase in the number of directly elected members such that they should constitute a majority over university and college representatives together, but would not constitute a majority when the Crown nominees were included. The working party saw the few Crown nominees as the only representatives of the public which the GMC existed to protect: it recommended a small increase in their number. Since the universities and royal colleges seemed unprepared to reduce their representation, the proposals implied a considerable increase in the size of the Council from 47 to 67 (see Table 4.1).

No precise recommendation was made as to the mode of election, but two alternatives were outlined designed to ensure that a wide range of practitioners would be elected covering all geographic areas, medical interests and age ranges, and both sexes. There was a marked absence of discussion about overseas doctors' representation.

Although the proposals were 'half a loaf' in the sense that functions had not been considered, the BMA RB at the ARM in the summer of 1971 accepted the working party report. The BMA representatives had included members who had been outspoken in demands for improved representation, notably Marks and Elkington; they, as well as their chair Ronald Gibson, were convinced that the best deal had been extracted on composition.

Table 4.1 Brynmor Jones proposals for the composition of the GMC

	Existing GMC	Proposed reforms
University appointments	18	18
Royal college etc. appointments	10	10
Crown nominees:		
medical	5	5
lay	3	5
Directly elected	11	29
Total	47	67

The GMC at its May meeting in 1971, as the president later reminded members,

> adopted a resolution that if the Government were satisfied that the public interest would be served by the implementation of the Working Party's recommendations, and furthermore that the recommendations would command sufficient support within the profession, the Council would be prepared to take such steps as might lie within its powers to give effect to them.
>
> *GMC Minutes, CXII* (1975), p. 4

Some ten months later, in March of 1972, Sir Keith Joseph informed the BMA that the government was prepared to present early legislation on the Brynmor Jones report. By that time, however, events had been set in train which were eventually to overtake that intention.

Fuelling the fire of rebellion

In December 1971 the GMC announced an increase in the annual retention fee—so recently introduced and still a matter of contention—from £2 to £5. The BMA council responded by reaffirming that its members should pay the retention fee but still on a year-by-year basis, and that the Privy Council should be asked to enquire into the GMC finances. The *BMJ*'s first leader (11 November, 1971) captured the mood: 'Patience Exhausted'.

Later it transpired that the Privy Council had no powers to investigate the GMC's finances, but the GMC did agree to having them examined by an independent firm of accountants, the choice of firm being agreed with the BMA. This, however, was not likely to be the end of the matter, for not only *World Medicine* and *Pulse*, but also the *BMJ*, pointed out the link between the cost of the GMC and its functions.

Meanwhile, campaigners were withholding their retention fees in protest: some who felt that they should not have to pay a retainer when they had understood on first registration that it was for life; others who felt the public should pay for the regulation of the profession, since it was in their interests; others who believed there should be 'no taxation without representation'; and a final group aiming for a more radical shake up altogether. The campaigners, who were variously estimated at 5300, 4000 and 2000—the true figure still being well buried—included two at least of the newly elected rebels on the Council, Dr Francis Pigott and Dr Katherine Bradley, both of the JHDA. Further fuel was thrown on when the GMC announced at its meeting at the end of February 1972 that it would ask government to amend the 1956 Medical Act to require all medical members to be fully registered. Although ultimately presented as a 'tidying-up operation' this was clearly aimed at the elected rebels. As *World Medicine* put it, 'GMC moves to unseat its JHDA members'.

The Tunbridge enquiry

Campaigners were not slow to take advantage of the increased hostility to the GMC which these two actions aroused. Their views were widely reported in *Pulse*, *World Medicine* and elsewhere. Critics of the GMC had expressed a great deal of concern about the GMC's functions as well as its composition. Anxiety was directed particularly towards control of advertizing, and other matters of discipline; registration, including registration of specialist qualifications and of doctors qualified overseas; and possible changes that entry to the EC would involve. In consequence of the pressures which these critics exerted, the BMA set up a working party on the functions of the GMC with Dr S. Wand in the chair. This reported in March 1972 and recommended further discussions be established between the BMA and the GMC, with an independent chairperson, if the GMC would agree. The GMC did agree to this proposal at its meeting the following May but somewhat unenthusiastically, making it plain that if an enquiry into the Council's functions were to be held, it thought it better that government should arrange it 'since the composition of any committee conducting an inquiry would need to be broadly representative and all interested parties, including the public, should be given an opportunity to give evidence' (Lord Cohen's presidential address, *GMC Minutes*, CX, 1973, p. 5).

A small working party with Sir Ronald Tunbridge (Professor of Medicine at Leeds University) in the chair was consequently set up in July to see whether, as a *BMJ* leader (11 November 1972, p. 315) later put it, 'the differences between the GMC and BMA about the former's functions [were] narrow enough to be resolved within the profession'. In broad terms the report suggested that they were: there was specific agreement that a statutory professional body should control basic medical education, registration and discipline. Not all critics shared this view, however. One group of those who were withholding their fees were doing so because they believed that the public, not the profession, should pay for the GMC. The Tunbridge working party, like Keith Joseph's intended legislation, was also overtaken by events.

The national press is alerted

By July of 1972, when the BMA ARM took place, the internal row within the medical profession about its control and regulation had well and truly spilled over into the national press. That ARM, in agreeing to the Tunbridge enquiry, had said that if the BMA and GMC could not reach agreement within six months then all doctors should withhold their £5 fees. The matter had reached such grave proportions that *The Times* (still under its former ownership and with its former stature in governmental matters) published a leading article on the GMC which suggested that an independent enquiry would soon become necessary. Supported by the view of the GMC recorded at its May meeting, Lord Cohen wrote to *The Times* saying that he was sure the Council would welcome such an enquiry.

Striking off the dissidents

Matters came to a head in November when the GMC voted to go ahead with striking off the dissident doctors who had not paid their retainers, all of them having already been repeatedly warned of this possibility. Lord Cohen and the Council took the view that it was unreasonable for the conforming doctors effectively to be subsidizing the rebels. The Council had agreed on the morning of that same day (9 November 1972) that it preferred to continue with the Tunbridge enquiry which it had started with the BMA, rather than having a public enquiry, so long as the committee could be widened to include a number of other bodies, such as the royal colleges, the medical defence societies and the universities.

The decision to erase, as Michael O'Donnell predicted in *World Medicine* (22 November 1972, p 5), made a public enquiry inevitable. This was so if only because the NHS would be put in jeopardy. Already some hospitals and health authorities had been asking practitioners to show that they had paid their fees before they would employ them. The NHS is required to employ only properly registered medical practitioners.

The Times devoted another leader to the GMC: 'Clapping Rebel Doctors in Irons'. The *Daily Telegraph* was also unsympathetic. Lord Cohen again wrote to *The Times*, saying Council would have no objection to a public enquiry. The debate which the BMA leadership had so earnestly wanted to keep in 'the family' was now out in the public domain—with whatever risks of further state interference that might incur.

Notes

1. I made a search of key medical publications from 1965 to learn something of the role they played and their view of how the dispute developed. I covered: the *British Medical Journal (BMJ)*, house journal of the British Medical Association (BMA); *The Lancet*, founded in 1823, with a world-wide circulation, a reputation for independence and no particular love for or loyalty to the BMA or the GMC; *Pulse*, a weekly newspaper, the oldest of the free circulation newspapers funded entirely by its advertisers, directed towards and delivered to general practitioners; *World Medicine*, also advertizer-funded but now no longer published, in magazine format and glossier than *Pulse*; and *The Journal of the Medical Women's Federation*. Other sources

used in this chapter in addition to those cited in the text include Jefferys and Sachs (1983), Klein and Shinebourne (1972), Stacey, F. (1975), Stacey, M. (1989a).
2. The composition of the Brynmor Jones Working Party was as follows:

Sir Brynmor Jones in the chair
Nominated by the Committee of Vice Chancellors and Principals (CVCP):
    Dr R. B. Hunter
    Dr H. N. Robson
    Sir Brian Windeyer
Nominated by the royal colleges:
    Sir Henry Adkins
    Dr Christopher Clayson
    Professor (later Sir) Norman Jeffcoate
Nominated by the British Medical Association:
    Mr J. S. Elkington
    Dr R. G. Gibson
    Mr J. H. Marks
Secretaries:
    Mr M. H. Barry (secretariat of the CVCP)
    Dr Elizabeth Shore (Department of Health)

5

The GMC, the NHS and the Overseas[1] Doctors

Issues associated with the employment of doctors qualified overseas—both problems about employing them and problems they were experiencing—were sometimes mentioned in the course of the professional revolt, but they did not constitute a central issue: it was later that the BMA began to take a sympathetic interest in overseas doctors' difficulties. The 1970 revolt was a revolt of indigenous white doctors about the way they were regulated. There was, however, a good deal of disquiet and discontent within medical ranks, and also in the popular press. Overseas doctors had become a very visible component of the medical labour force, to their colleagues and to the public.

If there was a public, as opposed to a professional, crisis of confidence in who was allowed to practise medicine in the NHS in the late 1960s and early 1970s, it was about the employment of overseas doctors rather than any particular objections to the GMC or the medical establishment as such. How far this was due to unfamiliarity with non-white faces in the doctoral role, chauvinism or racism, and how far it was based on difficulties experienced in practice, is another question. Patients, medical colleagues and nurses said they found difficulty in understanding and being understood by some of these practitioners: many others repeated hearsay. Doubt was also expressed about the clinical competence of some of them. Not all who came in were fully ready for service in the UK, but old imperial attitudes and straightforward racism undoubtedly fanned the flames.

NHS dependence on overseas doctors

The NHS during the 1960s had come to be dependent on practitioners recruited from overseas. The extent of this dependence was spelt out by the health departments in their evidence to Merrison. In the training grades there were 8000 young doctors qualified overseas, 42% of the total, most of whom would return home later. The health departments said (early in 1974) that, allowing for·the many doctors who returned home each year, maintenance of development of the NHS involved the annual admission of between 2500 and 3000 doctors born overseas. UK medical schools produced 2289 in 1973 . The number of overseas doctors practising in the UK, mostly in the NHS, was gradually increasing although the numbers needed were expected to decline as the output of UK medical schools increased (Merrison Report, 1975, pp. 58–59). In terms of the register, in 1938 about a twentieth of registered medical practitioners had qualified in Commonwealth or foreign medical schools, and by 1972 the proportion had risen to a third (GMC's evidence to Merrison).

The registration of overseas-qualified doctors

Arrangements for the registration of overseas-qualified doctors dated from 1886. *Temporary registration* had been first introduced in 1947 for doctors who wished to practise in the UK for a limited period only. When *provisional registration* was introduced in 1950 it applied also to the overseas qualified. Presumably in recognition of a felt need for the continuing presence of overseas-qualified doctors to staff the NHS, the 1969 Act had removed the 'temporariness' of temporary registration, i.e. those who applied no longer had to say they intended to leave the country within a defined period.

The GMC recognized some overseas qualifications for full and provisional registration as providing a standard (and, although not spelled out in the Acts, a type) of medical education deemed appropriate in the UK. The qualifications recognized were mostly those given by medical schools founded abroad by British doctors in the colonial empire where instruction was, initially at least, given in English. Recognition was associated with reciprocity, so that UK-registered doctors were entitled to practise in countries where reciprocal arrangements applied—this arrangement was clearly of mutual benefit in facilitating the mobility of medical practitioners within the Empire and later the Commonwealth. Government, through the Privy Council, was involved in establishing reciprocity with particular countries. The GMC arranged for the visitation of recognized medical schools, much of it informal; senior British doctors who visited for another purpose would report on standards and conditions. In 1973, 86 schools overseas were recognized.

Doctors who had qualified in such medical schools were accepted for *full registration* so long as the GMC could verify that they had clinical experience not less extensive than they would have gained in the pre-registration year in the UK. If they lacked this they could apply for provisional registration, but then they would be able to work only in house officer posts.

Overseas doctors who could not show that they were qualified for full registration, either because they lacked appropriate clinical experience or they held qualifications from unrecognized schools, could apply for temporary registration. Qualifications in some 70 countries were recognized for temporary registration. Doctors who were temporarily registered were licensed to practise only in specific appointments in hospitals approved by the GMC. Applications could be made to register for one such post after another.

Within the general rules the GMC had some discretionary powers such that the Council could withhold temporary registration if it received reports that the linguistic or clinical competence or the character or mental health of a doctor qualified overseas was in doubt. Its view was that it could not, however, require any tests to be taken (although, in the event, well before the 1978 Act was passed tests were planned and set up). In July 1973, 5799 doctors were temporarily registered under these arrangements. There was a route for these doctors to become fully registered: it involved obtaining the diploma of the Royal College of Surgeons (RCS) and the Royal College of Physicians (RCP), the licentiate of the Society of Apothecaries of London, or the joint qualification of the Scottish royal colleges.

In addition to the formal registration requirements the NHS had instituted a Clinical Attachment Scheme. The purpose of this was to help overseas doctors gain experience of clinical conditions in the UK and to help hospital authorities to ensure that doctors were linguistically and clinically competent.

Registration fees

Overseas, like home-qualified, doctors paid fees for registration. In 1973 the fee for full registration payable by an overseas doctor was £35; the fee for temporary registration was £5 for a period of two months or less and £10 for periods of between two and 12 months. This corresponded to £10 for provisional registration, £15 for full registration after provisional registration and £25 for full registration not preceded by provisional registration for UK-qualified doctors. The fee for renewal of temporary registration for an appointment lasting for more than 12 months was £5 a year. This corresponded to the annual retention fee for UK-qualified doctors.

GMC anxieties

Professional and public complaints led to GMC concern about whether the registration arrangements were adequate to ensure the competence to practise of all those it registered. The close links of senior British doctors with the recognized hospitals had loosened since independence had been granted to the ex-colonial territories; some schools were now teaching in the indigenous languages. Complaints reaching the Council claimed that some overseas doctors in practice lacked an adequate command of English and that some were not sufficiently clinically competent, although, as the GMC said, convincing evidence of these charges was rarely forthcoming.

Furthermore, the temporary registration arrangements were costly, time-consuming and annoying for the overseas doctors, as they also were for their potential employers—sometimes this resulted in doctors who were not registered practising in the NHS while the paperwork was being sorted out. There were also difficulties in the Clinical Attachment Scheme. Doctors did not always get the supervision they needed, and the reports which the GMC received as to linguistic and clinical competence, and which they used when considering applications for the renewal of temporary registration, were not standardized and were not always reliable or informative.

The Council consequently started an enquiry in 1971, consulting widely with other medical bodies. There were at that time no doctors qualified overseas on the GMC and none were co-opted. It is likely that on the basis of the enquiry the Council would in any case have applied to government for legislative changes. The events which followed the professional revolt overtook these plans along with others. In the event the evidence and the GMC's consequent recommendations were presented to the official enquiry, as we shall see in the next chapter.

At the time all this was taking place the overseas doctors were not organized. They came, after all, from a wide variety of places and by no means all shared the same cultural and religious backgrounds or medical education. However, shortly after the publication of the Merrison Report, realizing their need to organize to gain proper recognition, they formed the Overseas Doctors' Association (ODA)[2]. In practice it was composed predominantly of doctors from the Indian subcontinent. The Association's aim was to put forward the point of view of overseas qualified doctors and generally to look after their interests. Consequently, when Lord Hunt of Fawley became involved during the legislative process (see Chapter 6 'The Profession Transforms the Bill'), there was a body with which he could negotiate. The Association also had the effect of raising the consciousness of overseas-qualified doctors concerning the importance and mode of working of the GMC. It continued to be politically active and when Merrison chaired the Royal Commission on the NHS set up at the end of 1975, the overseas doctors were ready with their evidence.

Notes

1. The pejorative nature of the term 'overseas', referring as it does to Britain's former colonies, is recognized. It is used here because it is the term in official use by the GMC.
2. A strong impetus for its creation was the sense of exploitation young overseas doctors experienced, many of whom were employed a 'a pair of hands' without adequate supervision, training or other postgraduate facilities (see Smith, 1980).

6

The Merrison Enquiry and the 1978 Medical Act

Parliament acts in the public interest

Having authorized them to regulate themselves, the Houses of Parliament before 1972 did not pay much attention to the professions. However, the professional revolt then led to questions being asked, not because professional self-regulation might be breaking down, but because the NHS was threatened if doctors were struck off the medical register for failing to pay statutory fees. On 23 November, Sir Keith Joseph, Secretary of State, finally announced an independent committee of enquiry:

> To consider what changes need to be made in the existing provisions for the regulation of the medical profession; what functions should be assigned to the body charged with the responsibility for its regulation; and how that body should be constituted to enable it to discharge its functions most effectively; and to make recommendations.
> *Hansard*, House of Commons, 23 November 1972, Vol. 846, 464–465

Professional self-regulation unchallenged

It was plain from the outset that professional self-regulation itself would not be called into question. As Sir Keith also said:

> The General Medical Council is a body with a notable record of service to the public and to the profession. It is not contemplated that the profession should be regulated otherwise than by a predominantly professional body…

Sir Alec Merrison (then Vice-Chancellor of the University of Bristol, not a medical man) in accepting the chair of the enquiry committee accepted this limitation. The committee had 14 other members, of whom seven were medical. The general secretary of the Royal College of Nursing, one of the 'lay' members, was the only other health care professional. Five of the 14 were women; all were white and none of the doctors was qualified overseas. [1]

The committee quickly reaffirmed professional self-regulation. Evidence [2] suggesting alternatives, although discussed, was discounted. As early as paragraph 11 (Merrison Report, 1975), the committee state:

> We take the view that the medical profession should be largely self-regulated. The principal reason for our view is that we have no doubt that the most effective safeguard of the public is the self-respect of the profession itself and that we should do everything to foster this self-respect.

Further grounds were that

> the medical profession has been regulated by a predominantly professional body for well over a century ... a lay regulating body would labour under substantial disadvantage (paragraph 378, p. 133).

For similar reasons the committee rejected the idea that the Department of Health should keep the register and that lawyers should do whatever disciplining might be necessary. Regulation should be by a statutory independent body; the NHS machinery of itself was not enough. It was in any case weak, and there were private patients to consider. The BMA did not agree with its members who thought it should do the job and neither did Merrison.

The professional contract

In contrast to the Brynmor Jones and Tunbridge committees, the Merrison committee looked first at the functions involved in regulating the profession and second at what sort of body, and how constituted, should undertake these functions. [3] The committee started from the position that the essence of a profession is that it is composed of people who have specialized knowledge and skills which the public will want to use. The establishment and maintenance of the register of those competent to practise was central to the regulation of the profession. Regulation was 'a contract between public and profession, by which the public go to the profession for medical treatment because the profession has made sure it will provide satisfactory treatment', a contract providing mutual advantage (paragraph 4, p. 3).

Registration and education

Registration and education went hand in hand. A primary task of the regulating body was to ensure that those registered were competent and that uniform standards of medical education were reached by all those certified as qualified. Hence there was a need for a GMC with authority over the educational bodies to ensure the necessary uniformity.

At the time registration was in two phases: doctors who had passed a UK qualifying examination in medicine, surgery and midwifery and held a registrable primary qualification (such as MBBS) were eligible for provisional registration. They could then work in approved 'pre-registration' posts as house officers. After 12 months satisfactory service they became eligible for full registration.

The Merrison committee agreed with the GMC, the BMA, the JHDA and the Committee of Vice Chancellors and Principals (CVCP) that medical education required revision to fit it for the conditions of modern medicine. It was a continuous process which extended beyond basic undergraduate education and had to take account of continual changes in medical knowledge and practice. The committee accepted the evidence of young doctors, the JHDA, the BMA and others that the pre-registration year was unsatisfactory; a new approach and a new organization structure were needed. The universities, the medical schools, the NHS and the GMC were all involved but none had adequate power or responsibility.

The committee rejected the Todd proposals for general professional training as a way of progressing to full clinical responsibility. Identifying three stages of clinical responsibility—practice under supervision, independent practice, practice with responsibility at a high specialist level—it argued that there should be a corresponding three-tier system of education for all doctors: undergraduate training, graduate clinical training and specialist training. These should be defined in the system of registration and coordinated and controlled by the regulating body.

Successful completion of the graduate course should give the right to 'restricted registration'. Graduate clinical training, to make a clinician out of a graduate, would be the responsibility of the universities, but overall control would be vested in the GMC. Successful completion of this training would confer the right to 'general registration'. Specialist education should be a condition of independent practice, including general practice as a specialty. Specialist education could be developed from the existing work of the royal colleges and the joint committees on higher training. The GMC should have a role in its control and co-ordination, but the report left much to be worked out with the accrediting bodies 'in the give and take of consultation' (paragraph 135). The GMC should maintain a third, *specialist*, register, indicative in character.

The committee were not in favour of any sort of relicensure, but it did think the GMC should encourage continuing education. It wanted the GMC to be able to take more positive action to raise the standards of medical education and recommended legislation to give them this power.

Overseas doctors

The registration of overseas doctors was seen as constituting a special problem (see Chapter 5). Not only did the Merrison committee contain no overseas qualified doctors, but apparently no written evidence was presented to it from any of the overseas doctors themselves. Major evidence came from the GMC, which had rejected the idea of making foreign doctors sit a test like the US Education Council for Foreign Medical Graduates (ECFMG). Instead, the Council requested two main changes in legislation.

First, Council proposed that in future few overseas schools should have their qualifications recognised. Second, *temporary registration* should be replaced by *limited registration*, which would differ from temporary in that Council would have discretion as to the period for which registration would be granted (although there would be no residence time limit) and discretion also as to the range of employment which could be undertaken. Doctors should have a qualification which the GMC recognized as comparable to that of a UK-trained doctor. Furthermore, the Council proposed it should be given powers to test the linguistic and clinical competence of doctors qualified overseas. Provisions were suggested to enable a doctor to progress from limited to full registration.

The Merrison committee worked on the principle that only those overseas doctors whose standard was up to the minimum required of a medical graduate in the UK should be registered. Having sifted all the evidence which it received, including that from nurses, doctors, universities and the GMC, the committee reached 'the inescapable conclusion ... that there are substantial numbers of overseas doctors whose skill and care ... [falls] below that generally acceptable in this country, and it is at least possible that there are some who should not be registered' (paragraph 185). The committee blamed the division of responsibility between the GMC and the government for this state of affairs: the GMC had allowed 'its duty as the protector of medical standards to be compromised by the manpower requirements of the NHS' (paragraph 187). It recognized, however, that overseas doctors had made a major contribution to the NHS for which an immense debt of gratitude was owed (paragraph 195).

The committee accepted the bulk of the GMC's proposals, including its rejection of an equivalent to the ECFMG. It recommended the restriction of recognition as a route to full registration, the replacement of temporary by limited registration, and the imposition of clinical and linguistic tests upon those applying for the new limited registration. It also recommended that ways should be worked out whereby overseas doctors could apply for the proposed new specialist registration. The Clinical Attachment Scheme should be tightened and improved. The committee also recommended that the Department of Health should think about a training programme for doctors from overseas.

EC entry and the registration of European doctors

The effect of entry into the EC on the GMC had been around for many years. By 1972 the Council was already discussing the possible effect of EC directives for medical regulation. The free movement of labour throughout Europe, an important part of the Treaty of Rome, gained a particular significance in the discussions about the registration of overseas doctors. While nothing was yet certain it seemed likely that the UK would have to admit doctors registered in any of the member states of the EC. Linguistic problems loomed large in this connection. The potential contradiction in tightening controls on doctors coming from the Commonwealth—in practice, particularly those from the New Commonwealth—at the same time as controls were to be removed, loosened or modified on European doctors was obvious. The Merrison committee welcomed the mutual recognition of medical qualifications within the EC but hoped that means would be found of ensuring that the same fitness to practise rules would apply as apply to UK-qualified doctors and that 'incoming doctors are familiar both with English and with professional ethics and practice in the UK'. The GMC should register UK specialists for EC purposes (paragraph 218). The contrasts between the treatment of European doctors and doctors from ex-colonial territories was to become more poignant as the years went by.

Medical discipline and fitness to practise

Having dealt separately with the question of overseas doctors' competence to practise and what it saw as a GMC failure in that area, the committee turned to consideration of how the Council should ensure that practitioners named in the main register, known as the 'principal list', continued to be fit to practise. Whereas in the opening page of their report the committee had spoken of competence to practise, in this section they use the phrase in long use in the GMC, 'fitness to practise'.

During the professional revolt, many complaints were made by doctors about the GMC's disciplinary powers. Detailed criticisms were laid about the out-of-date handling of doctors charged with sexual offences; about advertizing, alleging the GMC was strict with rank and file doctors, while establishment doctors got media publicity with impunity. The handling of disciplinary cases was also criticized—the legal formality of the procedures whereby a doctor was literally put in a 'dock'. Furthermore, critics argued that the president was too involved in all aspects of the disciplinary procedures. He was the person who sifted cases to decide which should go forward to the penal cases committee, which he chaired. That committee then examined cases to decide whether to pass them to the disciplinary committee, where the president again took the chair. Some argued that, contrary to natural justice, the Council acted as prosecutor, judge and jury.

The GMC's own concern, as noted earlier, was that it was unable to deal competently and humanely with doctors whose mental illness—frequently in the form of alcohol or drug addiction—constituted a danger to their patients or themselves. Its power forced it to treat the 'mad' as if they were 'bad'. A doctor thought unfit to practise because of mental illness could only come before the disciplinary committee either after she or he had been convicted of a criminal offence or on a charge of serious professional misconduct. The Council had appointed a special committee to look into this problem in 1971.

The health committee

As to 'sick doctors' the Merrison committee found the case for separate machinery was well made and recommended the establishment of a health committee. The problem was serious: the NHS machinery was uncoordinated, insufficiently effective and did not apply to the private sector. The new machinery should apply to those doctors whose fitness to practise might be impaired by reason of physical or mental illness, as the BMA had suggested—the GMC's memorandum only referred to the mentally ill. However, Merrison rejected the idea of GMC-controlled local machinery and thought the NHS machinery if improved would be more appropriate. This seems to be in conflict with recommendations elsewhere that the professional regulatory machinery should not rely upon NHS machinery.

Discipline

Following from its decision about the propriety of professional self-regulation, the Merrison committee thought that professional discipline should continue to be handled in a judicial rather than an administrative way. The GMC, it said, while existing to protect the public was not a patients' complaints machinery. It was not there to punish doctors but to maintain the standards of the profession. Patients wishing redress should take a legal route. So the committee upheld the Council's powers whereby practitioners could only be removed from the register if they had been convicted of an offence in a criminal court of a kind which indicated they were unfit to practise or they were found guilty of serious professional misconduct. Were relicensure ever to be introduced, the committee argued, it could only supplement, not replace, the fitness to practise procedures.

Members of the profession had complained that doctors arraigned before the GMC after a court conviction were effectively 'tried twice'; wasn't once enough, that was all most citizens were subjected to? The committee were clear that the additional appearance before the GMC had to do with the special standards which doctors must be expected to maintain if the public was to retain trust in them. The GMC appearance was not a retrial; the trial had already been concluded and a conviction had followed. The GMC appearance was about whether conviction for that offence was evidence that a doctor's fitness to practise was seriously impaired or that professional disciplinary action was necessary in the public interest.

There were problems about the way in which the GMC learned about doctors who might no longer be fit to practise. The Council was heavily reliant on reports from public officials and others; some cases required further investigation. Merrison proposed that the GMC should establish an investigating unit which could follow leads and establish whether there might be a case to answer.

As to sexual offences, the Merrison committee thought the GMC were insufficiently clear as to the aims of their disciplinary procedures. The control of professional conduct must, they said, be firmly related to professional function. High standards of sexual behaviour were needed because of the trust that patients must be able to place in doctors, given the intimate nature of parts of their work. Sexual relations totally unconnected with practice, however, need not be of such concern. It was important also that the GMC should communicate its aims effectively. These arguments also applied to advertising.

Code or guidelines?

In response to demands for a code of practice to give doctors a better idea of what might lead them to be disciplined, the committee thought building up 'case law', as had historically been done, was preferable. A code would inevitably be too rigid to keep up with rapidly changing social and medical circumstances. The committee did, however, strongly recommend that the guidelines which the GMC issued to registered practitioners in the form of a 'blue pamphlet' should be considerably expanded: that would be the best way for doctors to gain an understanding of what constituted unprofessional behaviour.

The complaints machinery

The committee felt it important that the president should be the person to sift the complaints as they came in, but agreed with critics who thought it wrong for him to be involved in all three stages of the disciplinary procedure. It was pleased the present president had already reduced this involvement, restricting it to the disciplinary committee, although leaving his options open to preside over the preliminary stages at a future date. It was also pleased he had already abolished the 'dock', making the disciplinary proceedings appear more informal.

The *penal cases committee*, Merrison thought, should be renamed the *complaints committee*, but should keep essentially similar functions, i.e. to determine whether cases should go forward to the *disciplinary committee*, which should be renamed the *professional conduct committee*. The latter should keep its powers to admonish, suspend or erase in cases where a defendant doctor was found guilty of serious professional misconduct. It should, in addition, be given powers to make registration conditional in circumstances where a doctor's behaviour was not sufficient to warrant erasure, but the committee wished to retain oversight of her or him, or to limit damage she or he might do. It should also have the power of immediate suspension where it would be a danger for a doctor to continue in practice (orders for erasure ordinarily came into force 28 days after the decision was made to allow time for appeal).

There was some professional pressure for disciplinary hearings to be held in camera, rather than open to the public as was normal. The grounds were that a doctor's reputation could suffer from the hearing being reported and that 'mud' would stick even if she or he were found not guilty. Merrison proposed certain reporting restrictions until a decision had been reached and that only cases where the defendant doctor was found guilty should be reported.

Appeals

The Merrison committee reaffirmed that it was appropriate that appeals should only be on how the committee had conducted a case and should not be widened to question the judgement about fitness to practise. It clarified that the judicial committee of the Privy Council was the appropriate body to hear appeals. It ruled out appeal by complainants on the grounds that the GMC's task was to protect the public and not to act adversarily on the merits of a case.

Proactive about conduct

Merrison suggested that the GMC should have a statutory responsibility to promote high standards of professional conduct. There was a multiplicity of bodies involved—which the committee thought should continue—but since the powers of medicine were so great and still increasing, the committee felt that the GMC should be at the centre of public debate on the many serious issues involved.

Alternative practitioners

The committee did not think all treatment should be restricted to registered medical practitioners: that would not be practicable. However, it did think that the provision which made it an offence to pretend to be a registered medical practitioner should be strengthened.

The structure and composition of the regulating body

In its concluding chapter the committee reaffirms that the body which should regulate the profession, the new GMC, should be professional rather than lay-controlled. However, the point of view of members of the lay public could be available in discussions. The new GMC should be independent of both NHS and government and members elected by the totality of registered medical practitioners should have a dominant position. Given their understanding of the functions of the new Council and the close interconnection between education and registration, the committee rejected the proposals which had been made to divide the Council into two, one part to look after education, the other the register.

The Merrison committee settled the dispute about the size of the Council by proposing a larger *General Council* of some 98 members which would elect a much smaller *executive committee* of 18. It also proposed an *education committee* of 18. The General Council would be composed of 54 members elected in constituencies composed of each of the four countries of the UK by single transferable vote, a majority of ten over all other members. Thirty-four members would be nominated by educational institutions (e.g. universities and royal colleges) and ten members by the Queen in Privy Council. None of these ten should be medically qualified. To keep the Council independent of government and the NHS the appointment of Medical Officers of Health should cease, but they should attend as observers or assessors.

The president, elected by full Council, would preside over the executive committee. The General Council should also elect a chairman [*sic*] to preside over its meetings who like the president, would be an *ex officio* member of the executive committee. The General Council would be responsible for general policy and the executive committee would be responsible for implementing Council policy and be a source of new ideas (see Figure 6.1).

In considering fitness to practise, the Merrison committee had outlined their proposed structure for the relevant committees. As to committee structure, control of doctors' fitness to practise should be predominantly by

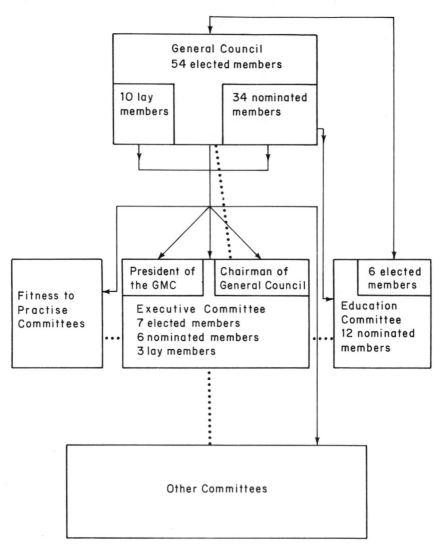

Figure 6.1 Merrison's suggested structure for the General Medical Council. → represents an elective process, ···· represents a co-ordinating function. Source: Merrison Report (1975), p. 137

those who were themselves in daily practice—hence the provision for a majority of elected members on all three fitness to practise committees. The complaints committee and the professional conduct committee should include some lay persons but Merrison saw no place for a lay member on the health committee, which would in their view make strictly professional or technical judgements.

Merrison's proposed education committee was important and likely to have increasing responsibilities if the committee's recommendations about education were accepted. On this committee no lay members were mentioned and elected members should be in a minority: educational interests should be dominant (see Figure 6.1).

Financing the Council

The Merrison committee found no mismanagement in the financial affairs of the GMC. Insisting upon an independent GMC, the committee thought that the profession itself should be largely responsible for its financing, although, given the use of the Council to government and public, there might be some governmental contribution. The Council should not rely on initial registration fees for its principal source of finance. Furthermore, the situation from 1960 to 1969 when doctors from overseas were effectively subsidizing UK-qualified doctors was 'unsatisfactory'. In 1961 fees from overseas doctors had amounted to nearly £31,000 out of a total income of just over £70,000. The annual retention fee was endorsed and should continue as a principal source of income: erasure should continue to be the upshot in case of non-payment after due warning.

From Merrison to the 1978 Medical Act

The GMC reaction

The Merrison Report came out in 1975: the GMC was pleased with it. The president, Sir John (now Lord) Richardson, welcomed it

> as an important contribution to the continuing evolution of the Council and its work ... main recommendations are entirely consistent with the views expressed by the Council.
> *GMC Minutes, CXII* (1975), pp. 11–12

In November the GMC submitted 56 pages of comments to Government (*GMC Minutes, CXII*, 1975, pp. 232–288). The Council was unsurprisingly gratified that Merrison had recommended that the profession continue to be regulated by an essentially similar body. It welcomed the electoral system proposed of four large territorial constituencies and the single transferable vote but did not comment on the proportion of elected members. Merrison's comments on finance were also welcomed, including the point that the increased functions suggested would necessarily cost more. The Council welcomed the health committee which had been its own proposal, and was prepared to accept the addition of physical to mental illnesses as coming under its jurisdiction.

The GMC was pleased also with the recommendation that it should undertake enquiries or commission research into methods of medical education and assessment. It agreed with the recommendations about specialist training and registration, including that it should maintain an indicative, not restrictive specialist register.

The GMC welcomed the recognition that it was not a 'patient's ombudsman'. Council thought Merrison was right not to try and impose a statutory duty on doctors to report the illness or misconduct of other doctors; that the Council should continue to take cognizance of criminal convictions and other proceedings against doctors which might indicate unfitness to practise; that there should be no code of ethics promulgated, but rather guidance should be offered in general terms; that the complainant's name should continue not to be revealed to the respondent doctor (although inevitably this sometimes emerges in hearings); that decisions should continue to be by simple majority on the disciplinary, or conduct, committee. Council would accept conditional registration, but noted that nothing had been said about the power to postpone which it hoped to keep.

The Council drew attention to those of Merrison's recommendations where it had already taken some action. Notably, it had arranged a discussion with leading members of major branches of the profession—to take place on 24 February 1976—on specialist training and registration. It had already made the temporary registration of doctors qualified overseas dependent on applicants successfully passing tests; already agreed that the president should no longer preside over all stages of the disciplinary process, although it did not wish to be tied by legislation as to which stages it would always be appropriate for the president to be involved in.

However, the GMC was defensive about a number of matters: its past record in handling the registration of overseas doctors, denying that it had given way to government's manpower requirements; its handling of the registration mechanism; and about the conduct of disciplinary hearings. With regard to the proposal that respondent doctors should be sent evidence in advance, the GMC thought the Merrison committee had not done its work properly—it should have taken the offered evidence from the Council's solicitors. The GMC agreed with Merrison that it should be vigilant about doctors from the EC, but complained that there were limits to what it could do because it was no longer a sovereign regulator, but bound by the consequences of the Treaty of Rome.

The Council was clearly opposed to the idea of an investigation unit; it thought Merrison was confused as to the Council's role and practice and as to the role such a unit might play. It opposed the discontinuation of warning letters, which it was convinced helped to maintain professional standards. It had not asked that the penal cases committee (or complaints committee—a suggested name it did not like) should have the power of immediate suspension and did not think this was a good idea. Nor did it think there was any case for enlarging that body. On the question of 'sick doctors', while it was pleased about the recommendation for a health committee, it was disappointed that Merrison had rejected the idea of local GMC machinery to back this up, arguing strongly against a reliance on the NHS machinery, not only because the latter was not working very well but also because it did not cover those in private practice. The Council objected strongly to the putative diagnosis of mental illness being revealed to the respondent doctor. It reaffirmed that it was not the Council's task to prosecute unregistered practitioners and, quoting a report of 1858, rejected any suggestion that it should get involved in such prosecutions.

On structure, the Council wanted the education committee to continue as a committee of Council rather than occupy the semi-independent position Merrison had suggested. The idea of a chairman of Council did not find favour and Council wanted to retain the present method for electing the president. It was opposed, too, to any shortening of the term of office from five to four years. Nor did it like the idea of the Privy Council being involved in the appointment of young doctors should the electoral process not produce enough. Furthermore the Council thought ten would be too many lay persons; seven would do quite well. On the other hand, contrary to Merrison, the GMC thought that a lay presence should be kept on the education committee and be made available on the new health committee.

The GMC resisted and was anxious about the proposals for graduate clinical training and the allied proposal for two years pre-registration. It spelled its reservations out at length and indicated that the whole matter would be discussed in the meeting on 24 February 1976. Here, as elsewhere, the GMC exhibited great sensitivity to the opinions and interests of other parts of the medical establishment and its need to take advice before adopting a stance or taking action. For example, while it was happy to take up the idea that the GMC should constitute a forum for the discussion of the aims, nature and content of medical education, it was at pains to emphasize that it was by no means the only relevant forum. It was anxious not to be seen to be usurping the proper role of the universities at any point, despite the oversight of education which was its responsibility. In another example, it would only agree to cease to use warning letters if the profession at large thought it should.

The response concluded by taking Merrison's point that the recommendations had been conceived as a 'logical and coherent' unity and saying that, although it would be easier to legislate on some parts than others, it would be a

> great mistake to legislate the parts of the Report dealing with the composition of the Council before those dealing with functions: the legislation which will be necessary for both purposes should be enacted in one Bill and on the same occasion.
>
> *GMC Minutes, CXII* (1975), p. 288

Two years before a bill is moved—and only half a bill

Despite questions and pressure from the GMC and the BMA throughout 1976, it was not until November 1977 that a bill was finally put before the Lords. David Ennals, for the government, had said in February that the profession agreed Merrison should be implemented; government accepted that the GMC should have responsibility for co-ordinating all stages of medical education and should maintain an indicative specialist register; it accepted in principle the need to change the mode of registration of overseas doctors; it also agreed that the GMC should be able to control the registration of doctors whose health endangered patients; and it accepted the majority of elected members. However, he continued, there were a number of issues still to be resolved: problems about graduate clinical training, about seats on the Council for the Medical Officers of the four countries, and about details of Council's composition (*Hansard*, Commons, Vol. 935–2, pp. 347–349).

The GMC fears that government might jib at legislating for the entire Merrison Report were justified, although functions were not left out entirely as Council had feared. The bill laid in November covered the reconstitution of the Council; doctors' fitness to practise; setting up the education committee to look after the Council's educational functions; and relations with the Republic of Ireland, the latter aimed to limit the powers of the Council to the UK rather than the whole of the British Isles now that Ireland was also in the EC. Second-stage legislation was promised for a later date (*Hansard*, Lords, Vol. 387, pp. 1147–1155). Government it seems felt it needed the profession's agreement before it could legislate more widely than this. Proposals about medical education were limited to undergraduate medical education; there was nothing about the registration of overseas doctors, nor about giving the GMC powers to offer positive guidance on professional standards.

The opposition, and especially medical members, considered the bill very limited. As Lord Hunt of Fawley said in the second reading:

> It implements only two of the five main recommendations of the Merrison Report; those concerned with the composition of the General Medical

Council, and its role in relation to sick doctors and their fitness to practise. The three other important recommendations of Merrison which have been left out of this Bill concern postgraduate medical training, ... the maintenance of standards, and the registration of overseas doctors.

Hansard, Lords, Vol. 387, p. 1166

The profession transforms the bill

Fortunately for the GMC, Lord Hunt of Fawley, a London GP who was looking for a topic area to pursue, took up this cause. He busied himself with discussions among all those parts of the profession where differences remained and continued to press a resistant government, putting down amendments against Government advice.

By January of 1978 Lord Hunt had achieved remarkable agreement within the profession on the missing recommendations. All those involved recall the way in which the telephone lines hummed early in the morning and late at night. At the report stage Lord Hunt moved amendments designed to turn the partial bill into a full-blown 'Merrison Bill'. As Lord Wells-Pestell for government explained,

during the last month circumstances [about possible professional disagreements] had changed dramatically ... and at an unprecedented speed. I have never known so much agreement to be achieved in so little time. The General Medical Council, the British Medical Association and the Overseas Doctors Association felt it so important that the Bill's provisions should be extended to implement Merrison's recommendations on a variety of matters that an unexpected consensus has emerged on these matters among those groups as to the form the provisions should take.

Hansard, House of Lords, Vol. 388, pp. 281–282

The government effectively capitulated, but with a good grace, and agreed to accept the amendments after proper drafting. Their problem had been the intra-professional disagreements. In the event some of the amendments were not introduced until the bill reached the Commons. The one 'Merrison' issue which was left vague was the specialist register—the one which affected the royal colleges particularly—but the powers were there to develop it when the 'time came'.

It was a remarkable feat on the part of Lord Hunt and the BMA, all of whose PR resources were used. Lay involvement in the debates in both Houses was minimal; no one challenged the rightness of the decisions being made by medical professionals. Thus was born the Medical Act of 1978 which doubled the size and extended the functions of the GMC. It was the profession's Act passed ten years after the professional revolt had begun. Much had changed in those years. The Act came into being in a very different climate from that in which its seeds had been sown. The UK had entered the EC, the overseas doctors had organized and formed their own association, the voice of the patient was becoming more insistent, and there were signals that the expansionism of the 1960s and early 1970s was over. The following chapters will look at how the reforms worked out in practice.

Notes

1. The membership of the Committee of Inquiry into the Regulation of the Medical Profession was as follows:

Dr A. W. Merrison	Vice Chancellor of the University of Bristol
Dr J. R. Bennett	Consultant Physician, Hull Royal Infirmary
Mr C. M. Clothier	Recorder, Master of the Bench of the Inner Temple, Judge of Appeal (Isle of Man)
Miss Margaret Drabble	Writer
Miss Catherine M. Hall	General Secretary, Royal College of Nursing
Mr N. G. C. Hendry	Consultant Orthopaedic Surgeon, Aberdeen Royal Infirmary
Dr D. H. Irvine	General Practitioner in Northumberland; Honorary Secretary of the Royal College of General Practitioners
Mr Ian Macdonald	President of the Council of Industrial Tribunals (Scotland)
Professor D. C. Marsh	Professor of Applied Social Science, University of Nottingham
Miss Audrey Prime	Staff Side Secretary, General Whitley Council for the Health Services of Great Britain
Professor K. Rawnsley	Professor of Psychological Medicine, Welsh National School of Medicine; Dean of the Royal College of Psychiatrists
Prof G. A. Smart	Director of the British Postgraduate Medical Federation
Mrs Jean G. C. Turner	Surgical Registrar
Mrs Mary Warnock	Research Fellow, Lady Margaret Hall, University of Oxford
Dr W. B. Whowell	General Practitoner in Leeds
Secretary: Mr B. Bridges	

2. Evidence to the Merrison committee came from: all the major medical bodies, royal colleges, universities, those responsible for postgraduate medical education, junior doctors' organizations, individual doctors, nurses, dentists and homeo-paths, the Patients' Association, and individual members of the public. In addition the committee talked to some 17 people: the president and other representatives of the GMC, the Chief Medical Officer for England, representatives of the Health Departments of England, Scotland and Northern Ireland, the Welsh Office, and spokespersons from the medical defence societies, university and postgraduate medical education, the British Medical Association, the Junior Hospital Doctors' Association and the Patients' Association. No original research was called for.

3. The Merrison report, 156 pages without appendices, was presented in April 1975 in six main chapters as follows:

1. Main principles and problems of regulating the profession
2. Education and registration
3. Overseas doctors
4. Fitness to practise
5. Other functions of the GMC
6. The regulating body.

7

Changes in the Composition of the Council

The Council I first joined

New members, especially those who have not previously served on a similarly prestigious body, may be impressed when they first come to the Council by the sense of dignity which surrounds it. This is associated with a formality and self-discipline, as I learned, which imbues all the Council's procedures. In their conduct members impose a high level of order and discipline on themselves, expressed in the punctuality and careful control of all proceedings. These characteristics which can at times carry a hint of pomposity, embody the importance the Council is felt to have which is first conveyed with the invitation to serve.

Suitably impressed, I felt I should arrive early for my first meeting. I was greeted in the lobby by a friendly member of the registrar's staff. In those days (1976) the inner and outer doors of the lobby were open and there was free access, but also always someone close by at the reception desk. Nowadays the inner door is kept locked, the lock being operated by a mechanism the staff control. I was met, welcomed and conducted along a corridor marked 'members only' and up two floors in an old but beautifully functioning lift to the members' common room. My hunch had been quite correct. Here members were assembling and exchanging news and views over coffee. This was no meeting into which one could sneak unnoticed at the last minute. When the time for the Council to convene was near, a warning bell rang to summon us downstairs to the Council chamber.

This room conveys by its style and arrangement the dignity and decorum which befits the GMC: the nineteenth century furnishings, the portraits and busts of former presidents and the stained glass windows bearing their coats of arms. 'What would they do when all the panes were full?' I sometimes wondered in the more boring moments of meetings. That would undoubtedly be a matter for grave consideration. The surroundings conveyed not only a sense of continuity with the past but also the importance of maintaining that continuity.

The Council then had 46 members who all met together twice a year in May and November. All gradually became familiar to each other, but the members one got to know well were the ones who served on the same committees as oneself.

The reconstituted Council

When the reconstituted Council met for the first time in 1979, it seemed a greatly changed body, doubled in size, from 46 to 93 members: there were not only many new faces, but also many more of them. The president had 'softened up' former members by discussing informally with those who were not closely involved what changes would have to be made. For medical as well as lay members, there were now more people on the Council whom one did not know. A most visible change was the physical reorganization which was needed to accommodate all these people; another was the presence of brown faces for the first time; a third was an increase in the number of women.

To make space in the Council chamber, the old mahogany leather-covered desks, with drawers in which to stow papers, and the heavy matching chairs were done away with. New lightweight seemingly plastic-covered tables and chairs replaced them. These were still almost the same red colour as the old ones, that full red common in dignified chambers, but the nineteenth century solidity had gone. A few of the desks were retained for particular uses—on the dais for example—as was the impressive nineteenth century presidential armchair.

Members could no longer all be seated for lunch on days when the full Council met. Instead, a buffet was arranged, committee rooms in addition to the dining room being used to cope with the numbers involved, which regularly included some officers who lunched with the members. Although less formal, indeed something of a scrum, the lunch, provided by a firm of outside caterers who always sent the same devoted team of waitresses, retained the high epicural standard the Council had become used to. The formal lunch continued to be served by waitresses in the dining room on days when members attended for committee meetings. Undoubtedly the increase in size meant a great deal more work for the full-time administrative and secretarial staff of the Council; this was not immediately visible to members, however, since the necessary changes in arrangements were undertaken smoothly so far as a member's eye could see.

The composition of the reconstituted Council

When the Merrison committee reported in 1973, the 46 members who composed the GMC were divided into four main categories: 18 of them appointed by universities and nine by royal colleges, 11 elected by the registered medical practitioners of Great Britain, and eight nominated by the Privy Council. The Brynmor Jones report (see Table 4.1) had suggested that elected members should be in a majority over those appointed by universities and royal colleges. Merrison, as noted in the last chapter, had suggested a Council of 98 with 54 elected members, 34 'nominated' members (from universities and royal colleges etc.) and ten members 'appointed' by the Privy Council. [1]

The Medical Act 1978 provided for the composition of the Council in its first schedule but did not indicate numbers. The schedule says that the General Council shall consist of elected, appointed and nominated members and that the number of elected members shall exceed the number of appointed and nominated. An order of the Privy Council provided that 50 members should be elected, 34 appointed by the universities and royal colleges and not more than 11 nominated by the Privy Council (*GMC Minutes, CXVI*, 1979, p. 3).

Table 7.1 compares the proposals of Brynmor Jones and Merrison with the composition of the first reconstituted Council. That 1979 Council was composed of 21 members appointed by the universities, 13 appointed by the royal colleges, and 50 elected by the registered medical practitioners.

The number of elected practitioners was less than Merrison had suggested, but was still a majority over all others. A bigger difference comes in the Crown nominees, where the GMC's wishes, not Merrison's, were followed. As to the dispute between the BMA and government about seats

Table 7.1 Alternative proposals for the composition of the GMC

| | GMC before 1978 | Proposed reforms | | Actual GMC 1979 |
		Brynmor Jones	Merrison	
Appointments:				
university	18	18	21	21
royal colleges etc.	9	10	13	13
Crown nominees:				
medical	5	5	0	2
lay	3	5	10	7
Directly elected	11	29	54	50
Total	46	67	98	93

The Decade of the Profession

for the Chief Medical Officers (CMOs), the Act said nothing. The compromise reached in practice was that the CMO for England should always be nominated, while those for the other three countries should rotate, one being nominated at a time. No specific provision was made for nurses, midwives, health visitors or paramedical workers to be represented: they, by definition, are 'lay'. Of the lay members nominated in 1979, one was a nurse.

The constituencies: electoral and other

Table 7.2 indicates the way in which the electoral constituencies were changed between 1976 and 1979. Representation of medical practitioners from the Republic of Ireland ceased as recommended, Northern Ireland, as one of the four countries of the UK, becoming a separate constituency returning two members. Wales was now separated from England,

Table 7.2 Mode of membership of Council members: 1976, 1979, 1984 and 1989 compared

	1976	1979	1984	1989
Appointed by				
universities	18	21	21	21
royal colleges[a]	9	13	13	14
Total appointed	27	34	34	35
Elected by registered medical practitioners in				
England and Wales[b]	8			
England[b]		39	39	42
Scotland	2	6	6	7
Wales		3	3	3
Ireland	1			
Northern Ireland		2	2	2
Total elected	11	50	50	54
Nominated by Privy Council				
medical	5	2	2	2
non-medical	3	7[c]	9[c]	11[d]
Total nominated	8	9	11	13
Total members	46	93	95	102

[a] Royal colleges include faculties and societies.
[b] England includes the Channel Islands and the Isle of Man.
[c] Includes one nurse.
[d] Includes one nurse and one pharmacist.
Sources: *GMC Minutes* and *Annual Reports* for 1976, 1979, 1984, 1985; GMC, personal communication, 1990.

returning three members, while Scotland now had six seats. England had 39 seats, making 50 elected representatives in all

Tables 7.1 and 7.2 conceal the detailed changes made, reflecting Merrison's proposals, to take account of the new universities of Leicester, Nottingham and Southampton which had no seats in 1976 and the cessation of representation from Dublin University and the National University of Ireland.

Eighteen universities had appointed members in 1976; from 1979 there have been 21 university representatives drawn from 19 universities. Of these, Wales and Northern Ireland have one each, Scotland has four and England has 13. Except for London (a federal university with a number of medical schools), which has three seats, each university has one representative.

As Table 7.2 also indicates, other educational bodies were treated similarly. The exclusion of the two royal colleges (of physicians and of surgeons) in Ireland and the inclusion of four new royal colleges (general practitioners, pathologists, psychiatrists and radiologists) increased the appointees of royal colleges from to eight to 11. Two faculties also included anaesthetists (now the College of Anaesthetists) and community medicine (now public health medicine). The Society of Apothecaries of London retained its seat.

Territorially, Scotland has three royal colleges and four universities; Wales and Northern Ireland have one university each and neither has a royal college; England has 13 universities and eight royal colleges, all London based. These differences retain some importance, but probably less now than formerly, since regular communications have been established among the colleges.

1971: Antecedent change

These may be important changes but there was an earlier transformation. The Council of 1971 had been notably different from its 1966 counterpart,

Table 7.3 Old and new members of the GMC in 1971 by mode of membership

| | Members on | | |
	Previous Council	New Council	Total
Nominated	6	2	8
Appointed			
by universities	10	8	18
by royal colleges	5	5	10
Elected	1	10	11
Total	22	25	47

Source: *GMC Annual Reports* and *Minutes*, 1966, 1971.

not in formal constitution but in those who took seats (see Table 7.3), a quite remarkable turnover. This was the Council when the 'young Turks' were elected, including those who were refusing to pay their retention fees (see Chapter 4, p. 36).

A younger Council?

One of the major complaints from dissidents hod been that the Council was full of elderly and out of touch people. 'The GMC: wild swings from an ageing fighter' was the *Pulse* headline of 29 April 1972. Merrison had proposed the introduction of the single tranferable vote to increase the representativenes of the Council with regard to age as well as to a number of other features.

However, the 1971 result suggests that the mood of the electorate may well be as important as the mode of voting. Before the uprising the electorate had not always used its votes on the side of youth or even middle age, as Table 7.4 shows. This table compares the dates of first qualification of elected members of 1966 with 1971.[2]

In 1966 nine out of the 11 elected members had qualified before 1930 (five had actually qualified before 1925). One may expect that the average date of first qualification will be more recent by about five year in each successive Council since members are elected for a five year period, although appointments are not necessarily for such a fixed term. The change from 1966 to 1971 is much larger than this. Elected member were the most recently qualified group (see Table 7. 5) while the royal college appointees, followed by the university appointees, were the most distanced from their house officer days. In 1971 elected members represented the post-war generation in a way that none of the other groups did.

Table 7.4 Date of first qualification of elected members: Councils of 1966 and 1971 compared

	1966	1971
Before 1920	1	0
1920–1929	8	0
1930–1939	0	1
1940–1949	2	5
1950–1959	0	5
Total	11	11

Source: *GMC Minutes* (1966, 1971); Medical Registers.

Table 7.5 Medical members of the 1971 GMC by mode of membership and date of first qualification

	Nominated[1]	Appointed[1]		Elected
		Univ.	RC	
Before 1920	0	0	1	0
1920–1929	1	5	4	0
1930–1939	1	6	4	1
1940–1949	3	6	1	5
1950–1959	0	1	0	5
Total	5	18	10	11

Source: *GMC Minutes* (1966, 1971).

Representation after the 1978 Act

Dr Gullick (1980) undertook an analysis of how the electorate used its votes in 1979. His findings shown in Table 7.6 suggest that the electorate followed the traditional status orders. The high success rate of medical school staff is notable; votes for consultants were in roughly the proportions in which they stood, but, according to Gullick (1980, p. 79), in proportions greater than their presence on the register. Junior hospital doctors did badly. Assumptions made by some that more elected seats would lead to more GPs on the Council turned out to be somewhat over-enthusiastic. Proportionately, GPs did less well (ten out of 49 getting in compared with 15 out of 51 consultants). They nevertheless improved their position among the specialties on Council as Table 7.9 shows.

Table 7.6 Numbers of candidates standing for election to the GMC in 1979 and proportions successful

No. and type of candidates	No. successful
51 consultants (in 17 specialties)	15
19 hospital staff in other grades (and in 10 specialties)	0
49 general practitioners	10
18 medical teachers (in 9 specialties)	10
5 community physicians	0[a]
8 others	4

[a] One medical teacher elected is a community physician and has been entered under 'medical teacher'.

Source: Gullick (1980), Table 2, p. 80.

Ageism

Veneration for age seems also to have reasserted itself. Table 7.7 suggests that the 1971 Council was more youthful than its successor in 1976. Furthermore, although the reformed Councils of 1979 and 1984 were younger than the unreformed 1976 Council, neither were as young as the post-uprising Council of 1971 had been. Note, however, that to be in your fifties is to be young in this definition.

Fearing that even the single transferable vote, on which they had relied as a means to a more representative Council, would not result in adequate numbers of young doctors being elected, the Merrison committee had suggested that, if at least eight young doctors had not been nominated for election, the Clerk to the Privy Council should himself be able to nominate enough such doctors to bring the number to eight. It would then be up to the medical electorate as to whether they voted for them. As we saw in the last chapter, the GMC did not like the idea and it did not come about. In practice some of the youngest doctors on the GMC in 1976 and none of the oldest were among the five medical members nominated by the Privy Council. After 1978 it was not possible for the Privy Council to attempt to redress any imbalance towards the elderly in this way, since only two CMOs were then nominated.

In 1976, as in 1966 and 1971, the royal colleges had sent the oldest group of members and this was still true in 1979. University appointees continued to be slightly younger than those of the royal colleges, but by 1984 royal college appointees were no longer significantly different from those from the universities. Elected members in 1979 were younger than they had been; in 1984 they were clearly the youngest group and had the widest age range, the BMA-sponsored members being outstanding in this regard.

Table 7.7 Comparative youthfulness of Councils 1971–1984: percentage qualified 31 years ago or less[2]

Council of	per cent
1971	48
1976	28
1979	34
1984	35

Geographic distribution: the prestige of London

If age was one of the problems of representativeness, geography was another. My analysis suggests that the main geographic effect of the 1979

Act, apart from the exclusion of those from the Republic of Ireland, was to spread representation rather more widely, if thinly. How far this may be attributed to the single transferable vote and how far to the increased number of elected members it is hard to say.

Within the wider scatter, the tendency for a disproportionately large number of members to live in the south east region was reinforced. The electorate favoured candidates from that region. While the distribution of university members reflects the distribution of the universities themselves, the increased number of representatives from the University of London and the fact that the Universities of Oxford and Southampton fall in the southeast region, added to its predominance.

A complaint heard from a number of doctors was that the medical establishment (from which the complainants felt themselves excluded) was dominated by particular prestigious London hospitals. Table 7.8 shows in which London hospital GMC members who had taken their first degree in Cambridge, London or Oxford were trained, comparing 1976 and 1979. The 'London influence' had declined a bit, but was still about a third of membership.

Table 7.8 London hospitals where members trained: 1976 and 1979 compared

	1976	1979
St Bartholomews	2	4
Guys	2	3
Kings College Hospital	2	3
St Thomas's	3	4
University College Hospital	1	3
Middlesex	1	3
St George's	1	0
St Mary's	1	3
The London	0	0
Total	16	27
% of all members	38	31

Specialities

Ideally, because the GMC seeks to regulate the profesion by consensus, all aspects of knowledge and practice should be adequately represented within it. Mode of practice, practice locale and conditions are relevant, as is specialty. Rank and file demands for better electoral representation partly derived from a feeling that general practice, the most numerous specialty, was, as it always had been, badly under-represented on the

GMC. Some specialists were anxious that their specialty was not well heard, being overshadowed by the 'big brothers' of medicine and surgery.

Table 7.9 shows the rank order of the specialties with the largest number of representatives in 1976, 1979, 1984 respectively; figures in brackets indicate the actual number. General practice took the lead from medicine and surgery in 1979, although still not reflecting the numerical position of general practice in the UK nor the numbers of GPs standing for election. Surgery has kept second place throughout while medicine has steadily dropped. Psychiatry fell out of the first five in 1979, dropping to eighth place.

A dramatic change is in paediatrics which from having no representatives in 1976 had seven in 1984. Paediatricians, whose specialism had developed rapidly since the Second World War, wanted a strong voice on the GMC, especially with regard to education. In 1980 the Joint Paediatric Committee of the Royal Colleges of Physicians of the United Kingdom and the British Paediatric Association (BPA) had written to the GMC president proposing that paediatricians should be directly represented on the Council. This was turned down, it being pointed out that they could put

Table 7.9 General Medical Councils of 1976, 1979, 1984: best-represented specialities by rank order

Rank order	1976		1979		1984	
1	Medicine	(6)	General practice	(16)	General practice	(17)
2	Surgery	(5)	Surgery	(12)	Surgery	(9)
	General practice	(5)				
3			Medicine	(9)	Community medicine	(8)
4	Community medicine	(4)	Psychiatry	(8)	Medicine	(7)
	Psychiatry	(4)			Paediatrics	(7)
5			Community medicine	(6)		
			Pathology	(6)		
No. specialties represented	18		19		21	
Total medical members	43		86		86	

Where members are in practice their specialty has been deduced from their post. Those members who are not in practice have been allocated to the specialty they are last recorded to have practised in. Academics have been recorded by the subject named in their post. In this table general practice is looked upon as a specialty and not as a locale of work.

Source: *GMC Minutes* (1976, 1979, 1984).

members up for election and that they were represented through university medical faculties (*GMC Minutes, CXVII*, 1980, pp. 70–71). The paediatricians had, after all, not yet achieved faculty status within the Royal College of Physicians but were organized in the British Paediatric Association. Failing to make a special case for direct representation, the paediatricians determined to gain places by election; they succeeded well, as the figures show.

The increase in the number of pathologists between 1976 and 1979—from two to six—was less dramatic but noticeable in the voice they brought to discussions. Pathologists were concerned about difficulties associated with the recruitment and training of medical students in pathology and an associated threat to medical pathology presented by the increasing employment of non-medical pathologists (see, for example, *GMC Minutes, CXVII*, 1980, p. 97).

Women

Before the 1978 Act, women doctors were not present on the GMC in anything like their proportion on the register. Merrison (1975) considered (along with other categories such as hospital doctors, GPs, young doctors) whether special places should be reserved for women doctors on the Council (paragraph 393) and, as we have seen, rejected this idea in favour of the single transferable vote.

Until the Todd Report of 1968 many medical schools operated quotas on the number of women medical students they were willing to admit, thus keeping their number in a minority; thereafter the quotas were removed and nowadays about half the medical students are women. Table 3.1 showed the gradual growth in the number of women registered medical practitioners up to 1971 and the slow reflection of these increases on the GMC. In 1976, of the three women members two were lay women nominated by the Privy Council. By 1990 there were 11 women doctors on Council.

Neither the royal colleges nor the universities sent a woman to Council in 1979 and only one in 1984 and 1989; the electorate is chiefly responsible for the increase in the proportion of women from about $2\frac{1}{2}$% in 1976, to 6.0% in 1979 and about 11% in 1984 (Table 7.10). Absolute numbers are more important than these small percentages. In this context ten women out of 95, or even eight out of 93, constitute a greater presence—and are a greater support to each other—than three out of 46 had been, when two of those were lay.

Despite Gullick's comments about the widespread feeling in 1979 that women should be elected, the electorate did not increase the proportion of women it voted for until 1984. The increase to five elected women in 1979

Table 7.10 Women members of Council and as a percentage of total membership

	1976	1979	1984	1989
Women elected	1	5	7	10
Total elected members	11	50	50	54
Elected women as percentage of electorate	9	10	14	20
Medical women as percentage of all medical members	2.4%	6.0%	11.6%	15.4%
Total women members	3	8	10	14
Total members	46	93	95	102
Women as percentage of total membership	6.5%	8.6%	10.5%	13.7%

Source: *GMC Minutes* (1976, 1979, 1984); GMC, personal communication).

represents no larger a proportion than one out of 43 (Table 7.10). The proportion has subsequently increased gradually, but still does not represent the presence of women in the profession. In 1985 about 23% of registered medical practitioners were women 125,390 men to 38,318 women (GMC personal communication, September, 1985). At that rate about a quarter, not a mere 10%, of the Council should have been women. By 1989 the proportion had risen to just over $13\frac{1}{2}$% of medical members, still an under-representation.

Overseas doctors

Before 1979 there were no overseas-qualified doctors sitting on the Council in any capacity. Whatever small contribution the Privy Council may have made to correcting the maleness of the Council, appointing two women before 1979 and three thereafter, it did nothing to correct its whiteness. Nor apparently was the GMC much worried about this. When a full (unreformed) Council meeting was discussing new proposals for the registration of doctors qualified overseas, I asked the president whether overseas doctors had been consulted. He replied shortly 'No, Professor Stacey'.

Paragraph 392 of the Merrison Report (1975) says:

We have said we regard it as essential that the GMC should be as widely representative of the profession as possible: which is to say that every member of the profession should feel that there is someone whom he [sic] can regard as fully aware of his point of view, and with whom he feels he can communicate without difficulty.

Table 7.11 Medical schools of origin of Council members: Councils of 1976, 1979 and 1984 compared

	1976		1979		1984	
	No.	%	No.	%	No.	%
Indian subcontinent	0	0	5	6	6	7
Scotland (4 schools)	13	28	25	28	22	26
Belfast (N. Ireland)	3	7	5	6	5	6
Dublin (Ireland)	4	9	1	1	3	3
Cardiff (Wales)	0	0	3	3	1	1
All English schools	24	55	47	54	48	56
All medical members	44		86		86	

Source: GMC papers.

However, among the examples of categories for whom special places might be reserved (paragraph 393) no reference was made to overseas doctors although the committee knew and acknowledged how dependent the NHS had become on overseas-qualified doctors. By 1972, they constituted a third of registered medical practitioners; in addition they made up 42% of NHS training grades. Nevertheless, no reference was made to any particular disability from which such doctors suffered in achieving a seat on the Council.

Until the 1978 Act only fully registered medical practitioners could stand for election. Merrison had suggested that this should continue. But the Act extended the vote to those provisionally registered or with limited registration (with a condition in the latter case of registration at least three years in the preceding four). This provision had been agreed in Lord Hunt's negotiations (Chapter 6). Five overseas doctors gained seats on the Council in 1979 out of 34 who had stood for election (Gullick, 1980), i.e. about 6% of the total, a small proportion in relation to their numbers in the NHS. Until 1989 overseas doctors only gained seats by election. In 1991 there are eight overseas-qualified doctors of whom one is a woman and one appointed by a university.

Organizational representation

Which organizations may control or have strong influence in the GMC is of real concern. The overseas doctors have gained these seats because they had organized into the Overseas Doctors Association (ODA) and sponsored candidates. In this they were following a long established sponsorship tradition. Apart from the 1971 election when the BMA did not sponsor any candidates because of the delicate negotiations with the GMC, the BMA regularly put forward a slate.

Gullick (1980) estimated that nearly half the elected members were sponsored in 1979 (see Table 7.12). Fifteen of the 39 BMA-sponsored candidates in England were elected; four of the ODA's 13 (the fifth overseas doctor elected for England stood independently)—the BMA had sponsored no overseas doctor, although many were members; three of the 12 sponsored by the British Hospital Doctors Federation (BDHA, composed of the Hospital Consultants and Specialists Association (HCSA) and the Junior Hospital Doctors Association (JHDA)); two of the Medical Women's Federation's (MWF) four. None of the three put up by the Medical Practitioners Union (MPU) was elected. To see how the single transferable vote was working Gullick (1980, pp. 80–82) followed through 'the 117 stages of the count throughout which the "inheritance" of later preferences of the eliminated are distributed to those still in the race' (p. 80). From this he worked out a 'solidarity index' of continuing support for organization candidates. He calculated that a 'solidarity index' of 20% or more (i.e. at least 10% more than found in random groups) 'would probably signify that members of the sponsoring body took positive note of their party list when voting' (p. 81).

Table 7.12 Sponsorship of candidates and numbers successful

Sponsored by	Candidates	Elected
British Hospital Doctors Federation (BHDF)		
HSCA	6	2[a]
JHDA	6	1[b]
British Medical Association (BMA)		
Consultants	8	4
Other hospital staff	10	0
General practitioners	13	6
Community physicians	2	1[c]
Others	6	4[d]
Medical Women's Federation (MWF)	4	2[e]
Medical Practitioners Union (MPU)	3	0
Overseas Doctors Association	13	4[f]

[a] Both consultants. One candidate appeared on the lists of both HCSA and MWF and was successful.
[b] A consultant.
[c] The community physician on the BMA list who was successful has been classified as 'academic' as his primary appointment is a university one.
Source: Gullick (1980), Table 3, p. 80.
[d] Two teachers and BMA staff members.
[e] One consultant, one teacher.
[f] Three consultants and one G.P.

The MDU voters were solidary if unsuccessful. The overseas doctors demonstrated the highest solidarity; 'no less than 89% of the distributed preferences of their successively eliminated nine colleagues were conserved by transfer to [the] survivors' (Gullick, 1980, p. 82). No calculation was possible for the MWF because the two successful candidates were both elected before their colleagues were eliminated (Gullick, 1980, p. 81). However there was a tendency for votes to go to women regardless of their sponsorship (index for all ten women over 27%). The difference between these two under-represented groups, women and overseas doctors, appears to have derived from a generalized feeling that women candidates should receive votes while the overseas doctors had to rely much more on each other.

Members of the BHDF voted to some extent as a group (39% overall), all members of the career grades—consultants and specialists—appearing more solidary than the junior hospital doctors. The BMA votes, hard to analyse because of its complex structure, suggest that the oldest established GP interest, institutionalized in the BMA's General Medical Services Committee (GMSC), showed the highest 'craft solidarity'. 'But BMA members spread their votes fairly widely over the list, to secure a high degree of conservation within the total group' (Gullick, 1980, p. 82).

The laity

The British General Medical Council is unusual among other similar medical bodies in including lay members:

> Since 1926, it had been the practice of His Majesty on the advice of his Privy Council, to include one layman [*sic*] among the five persons nominated to the Council. The original intention, for which Mr. Bernard Shaw claimed some credit, appears to have been that a member of the public should maintain a critical vigilance over the Council, especially in matters of discipline, and should 'represent the consumer interest'.
>
> Pyke-Lees (1958), p. 17

Regulatory bodies which include lay members in any numbers tend to be those like the Swedish (Rosenthal, 1987) which have been specifically constituted to replace medical self-regulation. Merrison rejected the idea of lay control, but suggested ten lay members out of 98; seven were appointed to the 1979 Council (see Table 7.1). A 'lay' member is one who is not medically qualified, defined strictly to mean possessing a registrable medical qualification or being registered with the GMC. So a nurse is not medically qualified, nor are any other members of the health care professions. When the Merrison Report was discussed on the GMC, I suggested the 'truly lay', i.e. those whose only relationship with medical practice is as a patient, should be distinguished from non-medical health care professionals, such as nurses, midwives, and therapists of various kinds, who should have representation in their own right; they could make a particular contribution to medical regulation distinct from both doctors and the 'truly lay'. Furthermore, doctors sit on the regulatory bodies of those professions; reciprocity seemed in order. However, this sugestion did not find favour.

Before the 1978 Act the Privy Council customarily nominated two politicians and a lay member of a university; from 1955 one at least of these was a woman. Practice changed after the Act, which laid down (in schedule 1) that a majority of nominated members should be lay, one at least from each of the four countries. The Council had not found the political members 'very useful' and they were dropped in 1979. Of the seven members nominated in 1979 four were from the Community Health Councils of the four countries; one was an academic member as before (I was reappointed in that guise); the then chairperson of the body which regulated the professions supplementary to medicine, an academic administrator, was also appointed; a nurse, the then chairperson of the United Kingdom Central Council (UKCC), the nurses' regulatory body, was the seventh 'lay' member.

Seven lay members out of a total of 93, compared with three out of 46 as previously, is a roughly similar proportion, or less if one is talking of the 'truly lay'. The Council has subsequently increased the number of lay members, first to nine and then to 11. This last increase, which the Council felt was 'appropriate', may have threatened the *overall* majority of elected medical members required by statute, hence the increase in their numbers from 50 to 54. In 1989 politicians were again included among the lay.

The changing composition of the Council

Political processes played an important part in the composition of the GMC in the 1960s and 1970s, without major statutory change. Furthermore, changes were made in advance of legislation by those who nominate or appoint as well as by the electorate. The 1978 legislation doubled the size of the Council and ensured a majority of elected medical members, thus increasing the number of GPs and BMA nominees. The introduction of the single transferable vote slightly reduced the average age, led to the inclusion of five doctors qualified overseas and increased the number of elected women medical members from one to five. The absolute number of lay members increased from three to seven, but not their proportion on the Council.

However, despite apparently radical amendments to the law, a number of conservative trends continued. The 1979 Council remained unrepresentative of the total medical profession in so far as junior doctors, women and overseas doctors were concerned. In this, and in the preference accorded to consultants over other types of doctors by the electorate, pre-existing tendencies reasserted themselves after the dust of revolt had settled. Despite the changes, the Council continues to be composed principally of an elite of white medical men.

The following chapters will look at how the Council is constituted and the way it works, and then examine persistences and changes in its structure and functions in relation to education and registration in the 1970s and 1980s.

Notes

1. Merrison inverted the contemporary use by the GMC of 'appointed' and 'nominated', although the Merrison usage had been what the Council itself used in 1966. I propose to use the terminology current in the Council itself at the time Merrison reported as this was what was also used in the 1978 Act.
2. Dates of birth are not always available, but dates of first qualification are. Although some few may have qualified as mature students later in life than the average, for most date of first qualification gives an indication of age and certainly of how recently practitioners had been throuh the medical educational system. These have therefore been used. They have been derived from the Medical Registers.

PART 3

HOW THE GMC WORKS

8

The Council, its Officers and Committees

My first meeting

The president opened that meeting in May 1976 by welcoming new members elected, appointed and nominated. I recall that in introducing me he described both my family and my academic career, remarking that he believed I had put marriage and family first—a way, I suppose, of making a woman academic more acceptable, now somewhat old-fashioned. He recorded with regret, and appreciation for their services, past members who had died. Finally he congratulated members who had had honours bestowed upon them (two knighthoods) or had notable achievements (one member had completed 25 years service on the Council).

Having formally approved the minutes of the last meeting (no challenge was made, nor were there matters arising) the Council proceeded to elect members to committees. The president made it clear that while some of the work was onerous in one way or another, it was the practice of the Council that members must accept the work to which they were called and that, in particular, the discipline committee was something no one liked very much but it had to be done. This was accepted by members (although I suspect there was some special pleading behind the scenes). In 1979 the new members were less willing to take this sort of ruling; they refused to serve on some committees and also tried to alter the GMC's previously arranged timetable to fit their own affairs (a BMA conference abroad was mentioned). Some members, myself included, used to the sterner discipline of the old Council, objected to this effort to rearrange our diaries on behalf of a particular—and newly arrived—group.

The structure of the Council, old and new

Before I describe the elections, let me explain the broad structure of the Council in 1976 and how it changed after the 1978 Act. As Figure 8.1

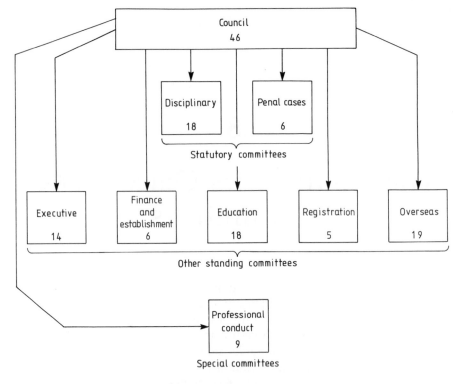

GENERAL MEDICAL COUNCIL 1976

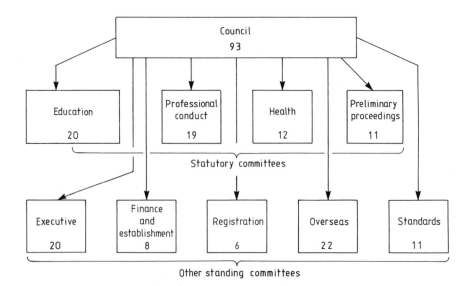

GENERAL MEDICAL COUNCIL 1980

Figure 8.1 General Medical Council 1976 and 1980

shows, in 1976 there were 46 members on the Council: two statutory committees, disciplinary and penal cases; five standing committees, finance and establishment, education, registration, overseas; and one special committee, on professional conduct, which had been set up in 1973. A previously existing standing committee on public health had been disbanded when the 1974 NHS changes had made it unnecessary for any medical officers in the health service to possess a statutorily recognized qualification in public health. Other special or *ad hoc* committees were set up from time to time in both the old and new Councils.

The enlarged Council met for the first time in 1979, but the new committee structure was not in place until 1980. There were now four statutory committees, education, professional conduct (replacing discipline), health (the new committee recommended by Merrison) and preliminary proceedings (replacing penal cases). The education committee, while elected by Council, has an independent status, following the Merrison recommendations (hence I have shown it larger than the three other statutory committees). There were in addition five other standing committees, executive, overseas, standards (short for the committee on standards of professional conduct and on medical ethics the successor to the special committee of 1973), finance and establishment and registration.

The work of the committees

The executive and finance and establishment committees served the functions of such committees in any organization. However in 1988 a working party on the GMC in the 1990s proposed the replacement of the executive committee by a president's advisory committee (see further discussion below). Until then the executive committee had been in principle responsible for the overall steering of the Council while finance and establishment looked after the Council's material survival. I will discuss the workings of other main committees in the following chapters.

Elections to committees

Figure 8.1 indicates the numbers of members on each committee. When I became a member elections for committees were held during the Council meeting in May of each year. At that time voting for committee members, like the medical electorate's voting for their members of Council, was by simple majority. At that 1976 meeting a although the committees were actually elected in that mode, an 'experiment' was conducted whereby three committees, registration, education and executive, were also voted for by single transferable vote in response to the Merrison Report. Six months later (November 1976) the executive committee reported to Council that the results of the two methods 'did not vary greatly' (no details were given or asked for): the committee recommended the single transferable vote be used from the elections of May 1977—a year before the Act and two years before its implementation (*GMC Minutes*, *CXIII*, 1976, App. XI).

Those May 1976 elections took a remarkably long time; I imagine they had always been fairly lengthy even without the experiment. Voting for some committees had to be done in stages: there were seats reserved in agreed proportions for elected, appointed, and nominated members and for the different territories (England and Wales, Scotland, Ireland). For example, elections for the penal cases committee started by voting for one elected and one lay member; then, in stage two, three more medical members were elected on a territorial basis. Executive committee elections were more complicated: in the first round voting was for three elected members of Council, three university representatives, two of the royal colleges and the Society of Apothecaries, one lay member and one nominated medical member. In the second round further members were elected on a territorial basis.

Merrison suggested some simplification, making no reference to territorial places, but even so the new method was going to take more time and space for staff to count. So it was decided that in future members should have the voting papers posted to their homes for completion, ready to bring to the Council before 10.30 on the day of the meeting. In 1977, under the new system, a list of all Council members was circulated, indicating who they were, their past service and which committees they were willing to serve on. This made choices a bit easier. By the time the Council had been reformed in 1979, sifting through data on all 96 members and voting in order for one's choice on each committee was still a formidable task. The president, later Sir Robert Wright, told me he had found it onerous—it had taken him all Sunday. It consumed my Sunday too.

Enough work for 93 members?

One of the anxieties expressed to me by Lord Richardson about the large size of the new Council was that it would not be possible to find work for all the members to do. With 46 members everyone was likely to find themselves on at least one committee. With nearly a hundred, and roughly the same number of committee places, not everyone would be on even one committee; those left out would meet only at the Council meetings in May and November of each year. This proved to be the case; members were heard to complain in the years after 1979 that some people were on large numbers of committees and others on none. The increased work of the Council in more recent years, in particular with regard to discipline (see Chapter 10), has finally resolved this problem. In 1988, 12 members of the

Council did not either serve on a committee or take part in the preliminary screening of health and conduct cases (*GMC Minutes, CXXV*, 1988, p. 346).

Sir Robert Wright introduced the device of a member's forum in November 1980 which was, he said, 'an experiment designed to enable all members to have an opportunity to discuss matters relevant to the functions of the Council informally but in public' (*GMC Minutes, CXVII*, 1980, p. 24). This forum was held in the afternoon after the formal business of Council was completed. The Council was in no way committed by what was said in the discussions, although ideas raised here, if they found general favour, might get onto the formal agenda later. As well as providing an opportunity for all members to join in and raise matters of concern to them, members could effectively address their electorates through this forum.

Officers of the Council

The president

Among the members the most important officer is the president. No sinecure this: as well as influence, the president has a great deal of power—which was much criticized during the professional revolt. Although the president's power has been somewhat modified since Lord Cohen's day, it continues to attract criticism from medical members. The president is by law chairperson of the fitness to practise committees, although he (always a man up to now) may appoint another member to undertake the tasks. Until its abolition at the end of the 1980s, he chaired the executive committee and is *ex officio* member of any committee he does not chair.

Historically the president chaired both the penal cases and the disciplinary committees as well as acting as preliminary screener, that is, the person who decides which complaints potentially involve serious professional misconduct and should therefore be forwarded to the penal cases committee. When Sir John (now Lord) Richardson became president in 1973 he changed that greatly criticized practice, separating the tasks. It was left to the president as to how he (*sic*) should divide them. After 1979 the offices of preliminary screener, deputy preliminary screener and preliminary screener for health were created (see Chapter 10).

In May 1980, before Lord Richardson's term of office came to an end, the executive committee started formal discussions, which were continued in full Council in November, as to whether there should be a fixed term for the presidency. The Council had historic memories of presidents who had held office for very many years: Sir Donald MacAlister 27 years (1904–1931); Sir Herbert Eason for ten years until his death in 1949; Sir

David Campbell for 12 years from 1949 to 1961; and most recently Lord Cohen, also for 12 years, from 1961 to 1973 when he resigned for reasons of ill health. Some members, represented by Dr Allibone, felt they would be constrained from voting for a younger man for fear he would sit in office for too long. With two exceptions, both in the nineteenth century, all past presidents had been over 70 when they left office. In re-electing Lord Richardson in 1979, given the new rule that members should not hold office after they were 70, Council had known he would only be able to serve until 1980. A proposal from the executive for a fixed term of seven years prescribed by standing order, but with the possibility of revocation in a particular case if a majority of members wished it, was passed by Council in May 1981.

During the Council debates on the tenure issue I noticed that possible future presidents were always referred to as 'he'. When I rose to ask, for information, whether a woman could be a president, the entire Council collapsed in spontaneous laughter. When this finally subsided, the president, Sir Robert Wright, assured me that she could be. There is no way of telling for sure, but I would guess the clear image of a president in the minds of the members was of a white man. The change that elected members were after was quite restricted, simply the possibility of a *younger* man. However, the working party of 1988 (see below) did envisage this possibility—at least on paper. For the first time when discussing the office of president, 'he or she' was used.

Sir Robert Wright, who described himself as a journeyman surgeon (maintaining the historic fiction of the surgeon's humility in face of the gentlemen physicians), had been elected president in a straight fight with Sir John Walton. The two men had been on the Council for about a decade, having been appointed to Council within a year of each other. Robert Wright, born in 1913, was the older by nine years; both had done committee work, but Robert Wright had served on more committees than John Walton. With Robert Wright's untimely death in 1981, Sir Denis Hill acted as president until fresh elections could be held. Sir John Walton was then elected without opposition.

Treasurers

Customarily there are two treasurers, the senior treasurer chairing the finance committee. John Fry (a GP and prominent member of the Royal College) did this from 1972, a couple of years after he was first elected to the Council, until 1989. Rank and file practitioners and the BMA had been concerned about the Council's finances (see Chapter 4). The treasurer is not a member of the executive *ex officio* but is commonly elected to that committee.

Chairpersons

Chairmen [*sic*] of statutory and other standing committees also have important positions on the Council. There was no formal chairperson's committee, although *de facto* they sat on the executive committee, but the president from time to time clearly consulted, or, perhaps more accurately, sounded out, his chairmen. Who shall chair the conduct and health committees is in the gift of the president, as has been mentioned. The education committee elects its own chairperson. In 1974 it elected John Walton to succeed Sir John Brotherston. The latter had served since 1970 and no longer wished to continue. John Walton remained as chairperson until 1982, when he became president. The education committee by now had become a statutory committee under the 1978 Act. The election for Sir John Walton's successor was a much discussed contest—discussed, that is, in breaks in meetings, during pre-prandial drinks or over lunch. The contest was between Professors Kessel and Crisp; the latter was elected. Professor Crisp was appointed to the Council by London University in 1977 and had served on the education committee since 1979. Professor Kessel was appointed by Manchester University in 1974 and had been on the education committee since 1977.

The president himself chaired the registration committee until 1979, when Mr Potter was appointed in his place. Mr Potter had been appointed to the Council by the University of Oxford in 1973 and had been elected to registration in 1978. Apart from two separate one-year stints on education, Mr Potter had not previously undertaken any extensive committee service. Nevertheless one had the impression that he carried a good deal of *gravitas* within the Council. Registration is one of the committees which do not publish their minutes, so the process whereby their chairpersons achieve office is opaque unless one is a member of the committee—and may not be very plain even then. There is a feeling in any case that the president may exert a strong influence in these matters.

A special committee on the registration of overseas doctors had been set up by the Council in 1971. The standing committee on overseas doctors was established in 1972. For a while the special committee continued but it dissolved after preparing the evidence for submission to Merrison. Robert Wright was appointed to the overseas committee when it was set up and was its chairperson from then until his death in 1981, when David Innes Williams, newly elected to Council in 1979, took over; he continued until 1988, and was succeeded by Professor Kessel, a long-standing Council member, as noted above.

Restructuring for the 1990s

A sense that the Council was not appropriately organized to handle the problems to be expected in the 1990s had led to the establishment of a working party in 1987. In addition to the chairperson, Mr Bolt, it had ten members, including one overseas doctor, two women and one lay member (a nurse, Dame Catherine Hall). It was charged with looking at the internal structure and procedures of the Council, communication within the Council, and communication with profession and public outside, and making recommendations.

The working party was conscious that its deliberations were taking place against a background of increasing public and professional scrutiny of the Council's work and an increase in private medicine. Its most important recommendations were to abolish the executive committee, as has already been mentioned, and that the Council should appoint an officer responsible for press and public relations, although the president should remain the Council's spokesperson.

The role of the president was examined, it being noted that the amount of work had increased considerably and that the load should be lightened. The number of fitness to practise committees the president chaired could be reduced and preliminary screeners (see the following two chapters) could do more. It was also suggested that the president could appoint a deputy.

The executive committee was to be replaced by a president's advisory committee. The functions of the executive to do with registration should pass to the registration committee; the remaining functions of the executive committee should be performed by the president and the registrar or by the president assisted by the advisory committee. This should be composed of the president, the deputy (if appointed), three elected members, two appointed members and one lay member, the last six to be elected annually by Council.

Rising costs were clearly a concern. Conferences, other than internal conferences, were to be held less frequently, and working parties to be kept small and to be sanctioned in advance by the finance committee, which in general was to tighten its oversight of committees. The working party was dubious about the communication value of conferences involving non-members and decided to place its reliance for better communication with public and profession upon the newly created public relations officer and a revamped annual report.

Democratic procedure?

Those used to bodies which are organized on Parliamentary lines or familiar with the elaborated procedures of the labour movement find the arrangements for running the GMC not only opaque but autocratic. The question of the presentation of minutes is one example. I have already mentioned that while the registration committee reports to Council, its minutes are not made available or published. This is true also of the finance and establishment committee, the special committee on professional conduct and its successor, the standards committee, and the overseas committee (although the minutes of its subcommittee which deals with some cases of alleged misconduct are—see Chapter 10). In committees, unlike Council meetings, there is no formal agendum for the presentation of minutes or their challenge.

Members commented to me that the people who got elected to committees always seemed to include those whom the establishment thought were appropriate—if one were left out there were powers of co-option. Appropriateness might be defined in a variety of ways: a missing specialty, a person deemed crucial to help develop a particular measure, sometimes a member, medical or lay, by no means a 'yes' woman or man, but with a particular point of view. There was some fairly overt guidance from the president of the kind 'Council has usually found it convenient that...', but for the most part how committee membership came about the way it did remained as mysterious to me as medical members told me it was to them. Comments of this sort continued to be made even after the method of voting was changed.

On the first day I arrived I was elected to the education committee (the academic lay member 'always was' I was told—although this is not the case in 1991) and also to discipline. The latter was not surprising: there were three lay members of Council, two were needed for the discipline committee and one for penal cases (see Chapter 9). Comments were also made about the way chairpersons from time to time 'emerged'—but how one was not sure. I noted above how some people had done long committee service before they were elevated and this might seem a reason for choosing one rather than another (the election of Wright rather than Walton, for example); but then again others had not been at all prominent in *Council* affairs before appointment (Potter and Innes Williams, for example).

The business of meetings is highly controlled. Many members commented to me that everything seems to be prearranged, including the decisions that will be come to. Where there is some disagreement, the matter will be postponed to come back again later, perhaps subtly modified. Where ideas the president wants to get across are not likely to be acceptable to all sections of a committee, they are raised orally to test the water (the issue of a specialist register in the 1970s was handled in this way on the executive committee). If a voice is raised with an idea for new action that finds favour with the chair or is widely supported, the best that may be achieved is a memorandum for discussion at the next meeting. The report will be prepared either by the officers or by them in consultation with a designated member.

It is not my aim here to analyse the GMC bureaucracy; that would be a fascinating exercise and would constitute a book in itself. Undoubtedly the sort of power which accrues to any permanent set of salaried officers in relation to a changing membership accrues to the paid officers of the GMC. A past registrar told me that how easy or difficult writing papers might be depended on how well one could read the president's mind—and presidents varied in that respect. Wherever the preparation for meetings come from and whether it is set up by the office or the president, the preparation is certainly extentive.

While some members, particularly the more radical, whatever sort of change they had in mind, objected to this control, others thought there was insufficient of it, particularly since presidents nowadays exercised a less dominating position than some had in the past. The image held by those members seemed to be of a leadership which guided Council as to what it should do and members who would obediently carry out those ideas and disseminate them. This was different from the more radical model held by those who felt that members should be fully engaged in the creation of policy and practice.

GMC presidents have to prepare their guidance to Council within constraints provided by the royal colleges and faculties, the universities, the BMA and other medical pressure groups, from time to time by the media, and also, importantly, by the government. Within such constraints the style which a president adopts, and the rules by which an organization is governed—and, quite importantly the way the salariat interpret those rules, when taken together—can result in bodies having a quite different flavour as to how hierarchical or participatory, secretive or open they are. By the time I had completed my service in 1984 the GMC was still to be found at the secretive and hierarchical end of the spectrum. Since the appointment of a press officer, the Council has an apparently more open, but no less controlled, even possibly more controlled, public face. Some members may have intended that the establishment of a committee to advise the president would go some way to reducing his power. It is unclear whether this is likely to be the case, although an increase in the influence of the salariat was clearly envisaged by the working party (see recommendation y, *GMC Minutes, CXXV*, 1988). Any reduction of presidential power is more likely to come from outside pressures on the Council than from these new arrangements.

9

Registration and Education I: UK-qualified Doctors

The regulation of medical education centres on the statutory registration system... The power of the registering body ... rests on its power to determine the standard of competence which it will require of those wishing to be registered.

Merrison Report (1975), p. 9

This chapter begins with a description of the registers the GMC keeps. Apart from mentioning the modes of registration of overseas-qualified doctors, the chapter deals only with the educational controls which apply to the registration of UK-qualified doctors. The very different mode of regulating doctors qualified overseas is discussed separately in Chapter 10. Having described the registers and the proposals for a specialist register, the chapter continues with a discussion of the education committee, its composition, mode of working and the 1979 changes. This forms a prelude to a consideration of a number of seemingly intractable educational problems the committee has faced over the last two decades. The chapter ends with a tail-piece about the 1991 government plans for improving clinical training.

The responsibility of the Council

The 1858 Act and its successors gave the Council responsibility only for basic medical education. The register which it established and still maintains relates to those basic qualifications. From 1956 the GMC has also controlled the post graduate pre-registration year. The 1978 Act gave the GMC responsibility for the co-ordination of all stages of medical education, but there is as yet no associated specialist register.

The registers

Nowadays there are two principal registers: the first, the main register (or principal list), of those who have been granted full registration; the second, of those who have limited registration only. Full registration is accorded to those who have appropriate qualifications from a UK university or certain examining bodies and have satisfactorily completed their pre-registration year and, since 1980, from any overseas university recognised by the Council. These include medical schools in Australia, New Zealand, South Africa, Hong Kong, Malaysia, Singapore and the West Indies (Williams, 1988, pp. 27–29). EC nationals qualified in the Community are entitled to full registration in the UK and may not be subjected to entry restrictions by the GMC, whether clinical, language or other tests.

Limited registration, which replaced temporary registration after the 1978 Act, restricts the doctor to hospital training posts and is only for five years (Wright, 1980, p. 15). Entry requirements for this register are that the doctor should have a hospital post and either have passed the language and clinical tests set by the Professional and Linguistics Assessment Board (PLAB) (which are discussed below) or be sponsored. Sponsorship has become relatively more important since I was on the Council (Williams, 1988, pp. 29–30). Transfer from the limited to the full register is possible, but the hurdle of the four-year residence restriction now imposed on immigrant doctors by the immigration rules of 1985 (Williams, 1988, p. 28) now has to be overcome. The Council reports, however, that transfers remain at 600–700 a year. All these arrangements particularly affect immigrant doctors from the New Commonwealth.

Temporary full registration may be granted to visiting specialists (Williams, 1988, p. 29) and a list of these is maintained; there is also a list of fully and provisionally registered doctors who are presently working outside the EC.

A specialist register?

To comply with EC directives a list of registered medical practitioners holding certain specialist qualifications is kept. This is not a register in the sense of those already mentioned and is not a public document. Practitioners may enter certain specialist or 'additional' qualifications against their names in the register. However, hitherto there has been no register of specialist qualifications and thus no guarantee that persons calling themselves specialists in X or Y have had any training in these areas of medicine. The issue, although not new even then, was much discussed in the 1970s, encouraged not only in the Merrison report, but also as a consequence of the UK's entry into the EC which required certification of specialist qualifications. In 1990, Council, after wide consultations within the profession and discussion on the executive committee (to my knowledge at least since 1976), agreed that qualified specialists could, but need not, indicate in the register any higher specialist training they have completed.

Entry to the registers

All those who wish to claim the status of registered medical practitioner must gain entry to one or other of the registers. Conditions for provisional and full registration are controlled by the education committee and for limited registration by the overseas committee. There is also a registration committee whose principal responsibility is for detailed matters such as the form of entries in the registers.

Control of registration and educational standards

In what follows I shall try to give some description of how entry to the registers is controlled, looking at the structure, responsibilities, nature and mode of work of the education, and in the following chapter, of the overseas committee.

The education committee

First impressions

From the outset I felt more comfortable on the education committee than on any of the other Council committees on which I served. The majority of members were educationalists and to that extent we shared a common trade, whatever may have been the distances between our disciplines and the very different ethos of medical schools compared with social science faculties. As John Richardson had said, it was 'convenient' that the academic lay member should serve on that committee. She might not know about medical education but she would know about universities and to this extent would have an understanding of the educational issues. This could possibly lead to sharper comment, and might also lead to a sympathetic but less critical stance and one less oriented to general public needs in medical education.

The responsibilities of the education committee

The 1956 Act required that persons registered should possess one or more primary qualifications, have passed a qualifying examination and have had necessary experience. Council had a duty to secure that the required standards of proficiency were maintained and that qualifications from all the institutions granting them met that standard. The Act defined primary qualifications as those granted by universities (e.g. bachelor of medicine/surgery) or other bodies (e.g. licences or memberships from royal colleges or medical societies often referred to collectively as the 'non-university licensing bodies'). As well as the necessary preliminary qualifications, the 1956 Act also required that, before being fully registered, a practitioner should have satisfactorily undergone a prescribed period of practice in employment. During this time doctors are *provisionally registered* with the Council, which had the responsibility for determining the prescribed length of what became known as the 'pre-registration year' or 'pre-reg. year' for short.

In 1970 Council deleted its responsibility to the education committee. Council's duties were then confined to *primary* qualifications (i.e. to basic medical education) and to the pre-registration year, which according to the Act had to be sufficient so that registration would 'guarantee the possession of the knowledge and skill requisite for the efficient practice of medicine, surgery and midwifery' (1956 Medical Act, Part II, 10).

Additional responsibilities after 1978

The Merrison committee was not the first to draw attention to the two important implications of the many changes which had already taken place in medical education and the speed of continuing changes in medical knowledge (see Todd, 1968). Doctors now needed specialist medical education before they were fully competent to practise independently; all of them also needed continuing education to maintain that competence. Following this line of thinking, the 1978 Act made two additions to the Council's responsibilities for registering primary medical qualifications: a general function of promoting high standards of medical education and responsibility for co-ordinating all stages of medical education. The latter new statutory responsibility was not matched by a statutory mandate, such as the requirement to register specialist qualifications.

The Act established the education committee as an independent statutory committee with specified functions. While it is the Council's business to set up and finance the education committee, now it was that committee rather than the Council as a whole which had to look after educational standards. The Council's powers of visiting, inspection and requiring information were transferred to the education committee. The Council was not particularly happy about the new status the Act gave to the committee. However, in practice the committee has worked much as it did previously, reporting its intentions to Council and taking heed of discussion on them.

The Merrison committee had been impressed by the informal control which the Council exercised through general advice and a pervasive influence on the educational system. The Act strengthened this aspect of its work by the requirement to fulfil the general function of promoting high standards of medical education.

Composition of the education committee

The education committee as elected by Council in May 1976 at my first meeting was composed of 14 people: five elected members; four representatives of universities and three from royal colleges and the Society of Apothecaries; one medical Crown nominee; and one lay member (see Table 9.1). The committee had power to co-opt three people and at its first meeting co-opted the two Irish members (one elected—a university person—and the appointee of the Royal College of Surgeons of Ireland. The committee sought, and gained in time for its next meeting, power to co-opt a fourth person—giving the place to a university nominee. It was then composed of 18 people, including the president, who sat *ex officio*: five nominees of universities, often deans of medical schools; five, including the president, nominees of royal colleges or the Society of Apothecaries; six elected members; one medical Crown nominee; and one lay member (see Table 9.1).

Table 9.1 Education committee 1979–1985: seats allocated to each mode of membership of the Council

| | | Mode of membership of Council | | | | | | |
| | | | Appointed by | | Nominated | | | |
Elected for year	Date elected	Elected	Univ.	RCs etc.	Med.	Lay	Co-opted	Total
1976–77	5/76	5	4	3	1	1	4[a]	18
1977–78	5/77	5	4	3	1	1	4	18
1978–79	5/79	5	4	3	1	1	4	18
1979–80	9/79	6	6	6	–	1	4	23
1980–81	11/80	6	6	6	–	1	4	23
1981–82	11/81	6	6	6	–	1	5[b]	24[b]
1982–83	11/82	8	6	6	–	1	5	26
1983–84[c]	11/83	8	6	6	–	1	5	26
1984–85	11/84	8	6	6	–	1	5	26

[a] In 1976 the committee had power to co-opt three persons in addition to those elected; in that year the committee asked for and was granted power to co-opt a fourth.
[b] Power was granted in this year to co-opt a nominee of the Councils of Postgraduate Medical Education, who need not be a member of the Council.
[c] In this year the right to vote for members in each category on the committee was restricted to Council members in that category.

Table 9.1 shows how the education committee was composed in the years from 1976 to 1984. Since, in 1976, the medical Crown nominee was also a member of a university, more than a third of the committee membership came from universities. The number of elected members was increased in 1979 and again in 1983. In 1979 the university and royal college places went up also, but not so in 1983.

Deference and university control

This situation did not change significantly until the 1978 Medical Act came into force in 1979. Then, as Table 9.2 shows, but contrary to any expectations one might have derived from the rhetoric of the reform movement of the 1960s and early 1970s, the proportion of university professors (quite apart from university members as a whole) increased dramatically. From 1979 until 1983, when a new mode of voting was brought in, professors constituted well over half the total membership of the committee.

It will be remembered (see Chapter 7, p. 75) that a tendency to defer to, have confidence in, the medical educational elite strengthened the nominated university group on the Council in the first round of elections for the

Table 9.2 Education committee 1979–1985: numbers of those elected and co-opted by Council to the education committee who were professors according to the seats allocated to each mode of membership of the Council

| Elected for year | | Mode of membership of Council Committee | | | | | | |
| | | Appointed by | | Nominated | | Co-op | Total | |
	Elected[a]	Univ.	RCs etc.	Med.	Lay		Profs	Committee
1976–77	0	3[b]	0	0	1	2	6	18[b]
1977–78	0	4	0	1	1	3[b]	9	18[b]
1978–79	0	4	0	1	1	1[b]	7	18[b]
1979–80	4	5	1	–	1	4	14	23
1980–81	4	5	3	–	1	4	17	23
1981–82	5	5	4	–	1	3[c]	18	24[c]
1982–83	5	5	1	–	1	3	15	26
1983–84[d]	4	5	2	–	1	35	15	26
1984–85	2	6	1	–	0	2	11	26

[a] Elected members of Council included no professors from 1976 to 1979; in that year they included ten; in 1984, four.
[b] The committee included a medical school provost in addition. In this, as in other committees listed in this column, all members were members of universities whether they were professors or not.
[c] Power was granted in this year to co-opt a nominee of the Councils of Postgraduate Medical Education, who need not be a member of the Council.
[d] In this year the right to vote for members in each category on the committee was restricted to Council members in that category.

reformed Council, ten professors being elected out of the total of 51 elected members. This confidence/deference also seemed to be shared by some at least of the non-professorial elected Council members. The second round of elections for the reformed Council was held in 1984. Only six professors were elected this time.

As Table 9.2 shows, those wishing to reduce the elite university influence on the education committee seem also to have been somewhat more successful in the new Council; two out of eight elected members were now professors. That summer I was replaced by Professor Ian Kennedy as the academic lay member. Members, however, apparently did not find it 'convenient' to elect him to the education committee (or perhaps he did not want to serve?). However, the total proportion of university professors on the education committee still remained higher than it had been in 1976. How the changes were wrought is an interesting example of the struggle between the three major groups on the new Council: the universities, the royal colleges and societies and the BMA.

The Merrison committee had recommended that appointed members (i.e. by universities and royal colleges) should have a majority on the education committee, in contrast to the Council, where Merrison had recommended an overall majority of elected members. However, Merrison had gone on to suggest (1975, paragraph 417) that within the Council the electorate for each category of member on the education committee should be composed exclusively of Council members in that category—thus, for example, only elected Council members would vote for persons to fill the six seats allocated to elected members.

This last proposal did not find favour with the GMC leadership, although, as noted in the last chapter, Council leaders were anxious about the shortage of committee places to go round its greatly increased membership. In a paper discussing changes which might encourage a wider spread of members among committees, the sixth variant suggested noted Merrison's proposal but concluded

> It is not apparent that this method would increase the distribution of places among members, and it would tend to introduce a fragmentation into a corporate decision of Council.
>
> *GMC Minutes, CXV* (1979), p. 415

Council members who supported the BMA's wish that non-university, non-college members should have a greater say in the regulation of medical education were not slow to notice the way the electoral system was working in favour of the university elite. In May 1982 the Council passed a motion from Mr Grabham, seconded by Mr Kyle, that the Council 'would welcome a higher proportion of elected members on the education committee'. In response the executive committee, although seeing a disadvantage in a larger committee, recommended an increase in the number of elected members to eight rather than a reduction in the number of university and royal college members. At the same time it was confirmed that the mode of membership of the president, an *ex officio* member of the education committee, would count and that lay members were to be included in the number of nominated members. Co-opted members, however, were not to be counted. These interpretations of the Act had the effect of ensuring definitively that the majority went to university and royal college members, which appeared to be the Merrison intention.

The reform was introduced at once; five of eight elected members rather than five of six were now university professors. This was not to be the end of the story, however. In 1983 the executive committee recommended that the 1982 arrangements should be continued. The May Council challenged this, the meeting accepting a motion from Dr Gullick, seconded by Dr Bennett, that for the year 1983–1984 the method of election recommended by Merrison should be introduced. This had the effect of reducing the professorial members from five out of eight to four out of eight elected members (see Table 9.2).

Establishing qualification for entry for UK-qualified doctors

The Council works through achieving and maintaining consensus throughout the profession. To ensure the standard of entry to the register the education committee works through the universities and the non-university licensing bodies. Those institutions educate, train and test the aspiring practitioners; the GMC is not itself directly involved. Because it relies upon the co-operation of those bodies, the Council has always been anxious that they should be well represented in all its deliberations. The Council's general educational oversight has to do, first, with the content of the education received, and, second, with the standards, appropriateness and organization of the qualifying tests and examinations. After the 1956 Act the Council had the power to appoint 'visitors', not themselves Council members, to visit medical schools to see whether the instruction and allied matters were 'sufficient'. After the 1978 Act Council members were themselves allowed to work in this way. From 1858 Council had been able to require information from the licensing bodies and to inspect any of their final examinations.

The content of education received

Knowledge of what is being taught is essential if any control is to be exercized. The subcommittee on examination returns kept in formal touch with medical schools and routinely received certain statistics and other data. However, these were not particularly informative about what really went on in medical schools. Consequently in 1973, when Professor Brotherston chaired the education committee, it initiated a thorough-going survey of basic medical education conducted by an expert (Richard Wakeford) and administered by the University of Dundee. The course this survey took and how the recommendations which followed it were drawn up illustrates well the close connection sustained between the educating bodies and the GMC.

The committee were informed throughout as to the progress of the research and senior member kept in even closer touch. In March of 1976, when the survey was 'near completion', a meeting was held with the deans and survey correspondents of medical schools (i.e those faculty members who had been allocated the task of providing the data), the researcher and senior Council members. This meeting agreed that

> the general section of the report and the school profiles should be checked by deans both for factual accuracy and with regard to any matters which a school might regard as sensitive and therefore to be treated as confidential.
>
> *GMC Minutes, CXIII* (1976), p. 142–3

The Nuffield Provincial Hospitals Trust paid for the final publication in September 1977.

These one-off surveys were institutionalized in 1983 when Professor Kessel, then chairing the subcommittee on examination returns, reported that the committee had decided to abolish the annual returns which made 'rather boring reading' (*GMC Annual Report for 1983*, p. 6) and replace them by a more detailed five-yearly enquiry, the descendant of Brotherston's first survey. The results of this inquiry became available in 1987 and suggest that the committee by then had a more systematic and realistic view of what its task in monitoring medical education required.

Recommendations by consensus

The GMC has for long offered guidance about the education received by doctors before they could be registered. From 1947 the Council had annually published *Recommendations on Basic Medical Education* for the guidance of universities and other licensing bodies as to what it considered the content of an appropriate medical education should be. These had last been revised in 1967. In May 1974 the committee started to think about further revision, but decided to wait until the survey was completed.

A subcommittee (composed of five professors, two college representatives and no lay person) was set up in November 1977 to work on the revision, but the new recommendations were not finally published until May 1980, the 1978 Act having added to the delay. Some updating of the survey results had seemed necessary. In this case the education committee, now chaired by Sir John (now Lord) Walton, decided to enquire itself of the deans and school correspondents rather than employ an external researcher.

The recommendations which finally emerged in 1980, like their predecessors, were developed in consultation with the licensing bodies for whom they were intended. The education committee organized a meeting of deans to discuss the objectives of basic medical education in February 1977. The subcommittee's report was ready for the education committee in November 1978 when a final version of the new recommendations was approved. This, with comments of universities, medical schools and examining boards, went to Council in February 1979 to be ready for the new committee of the reformed Council. The Council approved the draft, but this was not the end of the process. The draft was sent to medical schools and other interested bodies for their comments. So many were received that, in September 1979, the committee appointed a further subcommittee (with essentially the same membership as before) to look at them. The comments were incorporated into a further version in time for the November committee meeting and went to Council in November 1979, where only minor amendments were made. Council finally approved the revised draft in February 1980. The recommendations had taken account, not only of the comments of the educationalists, but also of the changes which the new Act was to bring into being. The procedures used had achieved two ends: maintaining close relations with the educationallists and ensuring continuity between the old and the reformed Council.

Continuities and changes in the guidance

The new recommendations (GMC, 1980) exhibited both continuities and changes compared with those of 1967. In this, as in other documents, the Council is anxious to guide rather than prescribe. The recommendations stress the freedom given to the universities to meet the recommendations as they see fit and their freedom to experiment, while letting the GMC know what they are doing. The 1980 booklet is more discursive, attempting to do justice to the new powers. Divided into two main sections, section A deals with the extent of knowledge and skill required for the granting of primary qualifications and the standard of proficiency required. Both of these are set out under a number of topic headings and stated in general terms (e.g. the basic sciences to be learned, but the blend of scientific and humanitarian approaches needed in practice). The patterns of pre-registration experience required are expressed in greater detail than previously. Section B, where the details of the undergraduate curriculum are to be found, starts with general comments which include the wisdom of encouraging special study during the undergraduate period, the advantages of integrated and interdisciplinary teaching, and the acquisition of clinical skills.

The two booklets do have quite a different appearance and feel in terms of their presentation, but all in all there is not so very much difference between them save those which stem from statutory changes, changes which one feels the authors of 1967 would have appreciated. Those apart, changes mostly reflect the changing conditions in which medicine is practised, e.g. the ageing population, new medical scientific developments such as clinical genetics and a greater recognition of the social and psychological aspects of medical knowledge and practice.

Basic medical education

In 1967 the Council had jurisdiction only over basic medical education, the object of which was

> to provide doctors with all that is appropriate to the understanding of medicine as an evolving science and art, and to provide a basis for future vocational training; ... not to train doctors to be biochemists, surgeons, general practitioners, or any other ... specialist.
>
> > GMC (1967), p. 4

The 1980 recommendations echo this:

> The principal objective of basic medical education is not to train specialists in any field of medicine or of medical science but to provide all doctors by the time of full registration with the knowledge, skills and attitudes which will provide a firm basis for future vocational training.
>
> > GMC (1980), p. 1

In 1980, as in 1967, five years is seen as necessary for undergraduate medical education; no reduction was possible (paragraph 10). (Paragraph 11 records the EC stipulation that six years should be the minimum for basic medical education but that the pre-registration year can count in this.) The system of clinical clerkships, whereby a student was attached to 'chiefs' in various aspects of medicine for a total of at least 18 months, was regarded as indispensable; the clerkships to be held in medicine, surgery, obstetrics and gynaecology, paediatrics and psychiatry. The student should live in hospital or nearby.

With regard to examinations, continuous assessment was the trend throughout universities in the 1960s. Within the limits of the statutes, which require some final formal examination in medicine, surgery and midwifery, continuous assessment was advised, rather than over-stuffed final examinations. The 1980 authors agreed with this, especially the use of performance records maintained throughout the course. By 1980 the qualifying examination was no longer defined by law as being in 'medicine, surgery and obstetrics', but left to the education committee of the Council to decide the extent of knowledge and skill, the standard of proficiency and the necessary patterns of experience required. Particular times for or modes of examinations were not prescribed in 1980; formal examinations of various types should be used. Students should have passed all the tests set before being permitted to sit their final qualifying examination: testing clinical skills was an essential part.

So far as preconditions for entry were concerned, the Council in 1980 continued to recommend a general educational university entry qualification, plus demonstrated competence in examinations in physics, biology and chemistry, with knowledge of maths gained either before or after admission. The importance of motivation and personality in student selection were noted in 1980.

Course content

Four fundamental requirements had been enunciated in 1967 (GMC, 1967): basic medical education should give the student knowledge of the sciences upon which medicine depends and an understanding of the scientific method (p. 7); a comprehensive understanding of man [sic] in health and in sickness and an intimate acquaintance with his [sic] physical and social environment (p. 9); the pre-registration appointments should complete the student's basic medical education and prepare him [sic] for the vocational training to follow (p. 9). Advice then divided the undergraduate curriculum into two parts: study of human structure and function and human behaviour; clinical studies and related sciences.

In 1980 advice was divided into three: the first as before, second, the clinical sciences (laboratory medicine), and third, clinical studies. Under the first head both editions stress human anatomy, physiology and biochemistry and the inclusion of human genetics and human growth and development, psychology, sociology and biometric methods. In 1980 specific reference is also made to pharmacology. There are few differences in what should come under clinical science and clinical studies. The 1967 version suggests pathology and microbiology could be started before clinical studies, as could pharmacology, while therapeutics should go with clinical studies. Clinical studies themselves were seen to cover medicine and surgery, obstetrics and gynaecology, child health and paediatrics, psychiatry, social and preventive medicine, and ethics and legal medicine. In 1980 an attempt was made to broaden the concepts of medicine and surgery, seeing them less as distinct disciplines, so that sub-specialties can be included. A wide range is listed under both main subjects although it is acknowledged that not everybody can do everything. Additions in 1980 to the 1967 list were general practice (reflecting the changed status of that specialty), the elderly, clinical genetics, radiology, anaesthesia, resuscitation and intensive therapy.

Ensuring the standards

It is one thing to indicate what the content and standards of medical education should be. It is another to ensure that they are achieved. Horder *et al.* (1984) are not the only people who hold the view that the advice given by the GMC is way ahead of much practice.

When I first joined the Council it only made visits to or reviewed the curricula of new or overseas universities. During my term of office the last of the new UK universities were recognized. 'For no clearly minuted reason' (Kilpatrick, 1985, p. 8) no inspections were made of the older universities after 1959 (Crisp, 1983, p. 32). In 1978, when I asked about this in open session, the president said the Council 'did not find it necessary' to visit old-established universities. However, in 1981 the presidents of the Royal College of Physicians of London, the Royal College of Physicians and Surgeons of Glasgow, and the Royal College of Physicians of Edinburgh wrote to the GMC saying they were doubtful whether medical students were currently being adequately trained in history taking and physical examination. In response the Council exercised its right to send inspectors to universities to oversee their examination procedures. There was some initial anxiety about this 'interference' in university autonomy, but the inspections were carefully handled; the reviews were entirely by peers—no lay persons were included (see Kilpatrick, 1985, p. 8). Although, on my reading, the inspectors' reports seemed to range rather widely as to how satisfactory they thought the examinations were, the education committee found them generally 'sufficient'. After I left the Council some questions arose about the sufficiency of the non-university licensing bodies, but since I did not see those reports I cannot say how they compared with the weaker of the university reports.

The survey of basic medical education had shown that the study of some subjects was honoured more in the breach than the observance. A glaring example which I commented on was the teaching of the social sciences, especially sociology. Rarely taught from a department of it own and given house room in a variety of departments, for example psychiatry, general practice or community medicine, the amount of time and the kind of teaching permitted was variable, giving concern to the teachers employed and their professional organization. In Oxford at that time, almost ten years after Todd, sociology was non-existent and in Cambridge it was not up to scratch. The Council had had a conference on the teaching of the social sciences the year before I joined. A number of further discussions were held at my request, but few resolutions achieved. Attempts from within and without the Council to ensure (a) that medical sociology was taught and (b) that what was taught under that name was indeed sociology as a sociologist would define it, were at the tine largely unsuccessful. This was an interesting example of the problems of integrating a subject into medicine which many of the 'chiefs' still considered not to be of the least importance or even downright subversive.

However, in 1985 the education committee set up a working party, with Professor Roy Acheson of Cambridge in the chair, to examine the uneven development of teaching in the behavioural sciences, general practice and community medicine. Enquiries were made and visits undertaken. The report suggested that:

> In some schools there is cause for concern because one or more aspects of such teaching have still not become established or else have withered under recent economic strains. The education committee has made recommendations based on these findings and has circulated them to all those involved.
>
> Crisp (1988), p. 5

The pre-registration year and general clinical training

The pre-registration year, introduced in 1953, constituted a year of all-round clinical practice by new graduates provisionally registered for this purpose. Upon satisfactory completion of the year a Certificate of Experience permitted them to be fully registered and to practise independently. The purpose of the pre-registration year was to complete the students' basic medical education and prepare them for the vocational, specialist training which was to follow.

The training at the start of the 1970s all took place in hospital. Many, especially GPs, saw this as inappropriate when the greatest volume of patient treatment took place in general practice and almost all hospital patients were referred by GPs. Although it had been legally possible from 1953 for health centres to be approved for pre-registration purposes, up to 1978 none had been approved, nor could pre-registration posts be held in other general practices. When I raised this in 1976 at my first education committee meeting, all sorts of (unspecified) difficulties were said to exist, but pressure to approve health centres continued. By 1979 health centres were gradually beginning to be used more widely. The irony was that just as soon as this had happened, some 27 years after the power existed, in

1981 the (then) DHSS wanted it repealed. Their reason was that, as a consequence of NHS reorganization, health centres as the Department understood them no longer existed. The lawyers suggested the regulations should be changed from 'employment in a Health Centre' to 'employment in a health centre' (*GMC Minutes, CXVI*, 1979, p. 330).

Dissatisfaction about the pre-registration year

The year was a source of all-round anxiety. In 1967 'almost universal disappointment' was expressed to the Council about it (GMC, 1967, pp. 9–10). The doctors complained that they were being used as pairs of hands to do chores and being overworked rather than being educated. In part the problems arose because placing medical graduates in posts to gain clinical experience involves the practising hospital consultants, the NHS authorities and the Department of Health as well as the universities. The Council in 1967 stressed its lack of control over aspects other than basic medical education which meant that it could do little to improve the undergraduate curriculum or the pre-registration year.

The *Recommendations* suggested that the universities should pay much closer attention to their graduates during this year. In the succeeding years the committee examined details of the placement and supervision of graduates. The placements were made within the medical system of training by apprenticeship whereby house officers, the graduates in training, were attached to a team or firm of doctors headed by a consultant, the 'chief'. This is similar to the pattern of clinical attachments in the undergraduate years referred to earlier. When the number of practitioners was smaller and the delivery of health care involved a less complex division of labour, the relationships with the consultant were personal and the junior learned by supervised doing. Merrison agreed with those who argued that this element was now frequently missing and should be replaced by more formal teaching. In the 1970s the education committee talked about whether the universities adequately fulfilled their responsibilities to their graduates; whether there was adequate consultant and other senior cover for the proper supervision and training of the students; and the relationship between service and education. However, I never heard the apprenticeship nature of training, tightly tied in as it is to the hierarchical structure of the medical profession, or the rota system, discussed in principle or detail in the education committee. Such critiques I heard among junior doctors, and groups of women doctors, and from more radical seniors such as those quoted. The activities of the education committee in my day assumed without question the appropriateness of the *mode* of learning.

After a GMC conference in 1972 on the pre-registration year, the education committee prepared a code of good practice. The draft was circulated for comment to medical schools, the postgraduate councils and the government health departments, modified, and finally published in 1974.

Anxieties continued, so in 1976 Richard Wakeford, who had undertaken the survey of basic medical education, was asked to survey (in conjunction with the education committee) the extent to which universities were able to comply with the 1974 code of good practice. A further conference, in February 1978, to discuss the replies concluded that the

> principal objective of the pre-registration year was one of learning by service rather than through formal programmes of postgraduate training.

It also concluded that the quality of experience offered had improved through increasing implementation of the code of good practice,

> though the situation was by no means perfect and some appointments were less satisfactory than others.
>
> Walton (1979)

Nevertheless, in 1977 McManus *et al.* (1977) referred to the year as 'chaos by consensus'.

Interface with the NHS

A shortage of approved house officer posts for graduates in their pre-registration year was reported to the education committee in May 1974. The question was how to make enough high-quality posts available in the next five to ten years to cope with the expected increase in the number of graduates. This was discussed at a GMC conference in February 1975 at which the second topic was the GMC recommendation that graduation dates should be synchronized. This was agreed as well as synchronizing the starting dates for the pre-registration year to facilitate a better use of posts. The general agreement was reported to the deans. Only a minority of universities remained out of line. The University of Cambridge was slow to fall in: the unusual step was taken in 1977 of calling three represpresentatives from Cambridge to meet the education committee to discuss why they had not complied.

A solution to the projected shortage of pre-registration posts depended upon the (then) DHSS. The Department was represented at the 1975 conference, after which letters passed between representatives of the GMC and the Department. They met that summer. By 1976 the GMC felt the matter was urgent—more new graduates would soon be out. Another meeting was held. The Department then agreed to take urgent action and set up that year a pre-registration house officer working group on which Sir John (now Lord) Walton sat as chairperson of the education committee and about which he gave oral reports to the committee.

The unity of all stages of medical education

The 1967 *Recommendations on Basic Medical Education* (GMC, 1967) had stressed that medical education is a continuing process

> which starts with premedical studies and continues through pre-clinical, clinical and pre-registration studies towards vocational training for a particular career.

There were four periods: premedical studies; basic medical education (including preclinical, clinical and pre-registration); vocational training; continuing education. Medical schools were advised to think about leaving out of the conventional subjects of anatomy, physiology and biochemistry, and also from the clinical subjects, what should more properly come under the head of specialist training; encouraging students to think rather than cramming facts.

The Merrison Report picked up this problem of continuity and concluded that the existing divisions were inappropriate, recommending replacing the pre-registration year by an extended period of graduate clinical training before specialization. Following the president's (Lord Richardson) policy of responding fully to the report and preparing for any Subsequent legislation, this suggestion was discussed—along with others of Merrison's educational proposals—at a GMC conference in February 1976.

The new responsibilities

In 1978 the GMC held a further conference on the pre-registration year. By now the new educational role of the GMC was becoming clear. Previously the Council's only statutory functions in relation to the pre-registration year were to make regulations prescribing the total length of the training, how long should be spent in each of medicine and surgery respectively, and the form of the certificate of experience which the doctor could obtain at the end. These regulations were proscriptive—unlike the recommendations and the code. Now the committee's powers were extended. The committee would have a new function

> to determine patterns of experience suitable for giving to young graduates general clinical training during this period ... to appoint persons to visit

hospitals which have been approved for preregistration service, and ...
powers to notify a university if ... an approved hospital does not provide the
required experience, or ... a combination of posts accepted by the university
... is unsuitable [in which case] the university is to have regard to the Council's opinion. But the Act leaves with the universities the primary responsibility for supervising the pre-registration year and increases their discretion
to withhold a certificate of experience from a graduate ...

GMC Annual Report for 1978, p. 8

The view that graduate clinical training should cover two years and
include formal education as well as the gathering of experience did not
'emerge' from the 1978 conference. It decided to keep the one year, to keep
it practical and to rely on informal instruction. The committee continued
to resist the introduction of formal training. Neither the 1968 Todd
proposals, nor those of Merrison for some form of general professional
training, found favour.

In 1984 Professor Crisp, then chairperson of the education committee
which was beginning to discuss 'general clinical training' (as the 'pre-reg.
year' was now called), explained the resistance to change as partly caused
by medical schools

who foresaw that their carefully developed and cherished curricula would be
eroded if graduation occurred earlier, and this just at a time when they were
attempting to do justice to 'newer' subjects and to forms of integrated
teaching ...

GMC Annual Report for 1984, p. 5

Even as the education committee published its revised recommendations
on basic medical education in 1980, derived from the surveys of the mid-
1970s and the subsequent consultations, it was aware that all was not well
with undergraduate medical education just as it was not well with the pre-
registration year. The overcrowding of the undergraduate curriculum was
in large part caused by the fragmentation of medical education; some of the
troubles of the pre-reg. year derived from the same source and from the
vested interests of all the educational bodies concerned. The committee
now turned its attention to exercizing its new responsibility 'to co-ordinate
all stages of medical education' as a first step in the resolution of these
problems.

However, in 1987 when the committee issued recommendations on basic
specialist training (see below) it also issued further recommendations on
general clinical training (GMC, 1987b). This gave more detailed guidance
about the pre-reg. year than the 1980 recommendations on basic medical
education had done. Specifically the new recommendations drew attention
to the need for educational supervisors for each appointment, responsible

for guiding the trainee's work and watching her or his progress; the trainee would usually have two and should not have more than four supervisors during the year. The universities would be responsible for approving hospitals or health centres and recognizing posts. The Council set great store on a short final section which picked up the theme of *The Recommendations on the Training of Specialists* (GMC, 1987a), namely the need for general professional training to continue after full registration.

Post-registration education: the co-ordination of all stages

In regulating undergraduate medical education the education committee and the Council had for many years been accustomed to work with the universities and other licensing bodies. They now needed to work with all the royal colleges, the faculties and the many other bodies involved with postgraduate medical education. Just how many there were and how complex the postgraduate arrangements had become is clear in Robin Dowie's survey published in 1987 (Dowie, 1987).

The first move was discussion within Council about how best to establish relationships with all these bodies similar to those which the Council had with the universities in the regulation of undergraduate education. It set up an all-medical subcommittee to take the matter further:

> By the beginning of 1982 meetings had been held with representatives of royal colleges and faculties and of the joint higher training committees, with representatives of the councils for postgraduate medical education and with postgraduate deans, with the British Medical Association and with representatives of junior doctors, women doctors and overseas qualified doctors, and with regional medical officers.
>
> Walton (1982), p. 6

All consulted supported the education committee's intention to exercise its co-ordinating function, reinforced at a conference the committee called in 1982 which also accepted that it should now begin to apply to postgraduate education the methods used in relation to undergraduate education. A consensus also emerged at the conference that the first task should be to look at general professional training, the stage which immediately follows the pre-registration year but which is not at all standardized, varying greatly from specialty to specialty as to what is included and what it is called.

In the course of its deliberations the committee moved from this concept to that of 'basic specialist training'—a change that was more than semantic. It signalled that the committee had turned away from the idea of a general professional training including formal instruction. That proposal, as well as improving the pre-reg. year, was intended to take the cramming of facts out of undergraduate medical education. Then the universities could educate rather than train in the knowledge that a further stage of all-round general medical education would follow for doctors not yet committed to a specialty. The committee

> had taken the view that it would be undesirable at present to consider encroaching upon the time devoted to undergraduate medical education in order to afford time for graduate clinical training [i.e. what happens in the pre-registration year] as proposed by Merrison.
>
> *GMC Minutes*, CXX, (1983), pp. 256

The committee was thinking of a period of training basic to specialization to follow full registration. In the document *Basic Specialist Training*, published and circulated to all interested parties in 1983, the committee stressed the importance of the doctor gaining an appreciation of medicine wider than her or his chosen specialty and, for those not committed to a specialty by the end of their pre-reg. year, of having an opportunity for broad study. The committee thought there was enough common ground among the requirements of most royal colleges and faculties for all doctors to study some common element.

This publication drew many comments from the profession which were discussed by Council and the relevant committees in 1984. Among the critical comments was an open letter from John Horder and others (Horder *et al*. 1984). Taking the pre-registration year and the first period of specialization together, the authors claimed this middle period of medical education had been undefined and unorganized for so long that there was great confusion; the goal of basic specialist training pointed in precisely the opposite direction to what they believed was needed, namely general professional training uncommitted as yet to any specialism. The GMC proposal would do nothing to help universities to follow the GMC's own 1980 recommendations, the authors claimed; a major opportunity to free up undergraduate education and to improve (indeed restore) the all-round clinical calibre of UK doctors was being missed.

The committee, however, heeded the commentators who supported the view that

> the acquisition by young doctors of experience in specialties other than their own chosen principal specialty should not become obligatory but was nevertheless desirable.

But the committee took note of those who said the arrangements for general clinical training (the pre-reg. year) should be examined 'including means whereby a broader training might be given in the period immediately after graduation' (*GMC Minutes*, CXXI, 1984, pp. 64, 65). In 1984 it initiated a study of medical education as a whole. In relation to this the committee proposed to enquire of the royal colleges and other relevant bodies what were their objectives in specialty training and their arrangements for maintaining the educational standards of doctors in independent practice.

The training of specialists

By 1987 the committee were ready with their *Recommendations on the Training of Specialists* (GMC, 1987a). This is a 26-page pamphlet with a further 53 pages of closely written detail concerning all the present arrangements for general professional and higher specialist training and a fold-out tabulation of the relevant regulations. The data for the last two parts were provided by the joint higher training committees and the royal colleges. There is not space here to discuss this miscellany; readers interested in these details are referred to Dowie's survey (1987) and the annexes to the *Recommendations*.

The recommendations were intended to complement and co-ordinate those of the many training bodies already in the field; they were not intended to restrict their freedom to continue to develop their own programmes of training and assessment. The GMC recommendations were designed to fill gaps. Given the confusion of terminology, the following definitions were laid out at the outset (pp. 2–3):

1. *Basic medical education* includes undergraduate medical education and general clinical training (the pre-reg. year) and concludes with full registration;
2. *Basic specialist training* occupies the following two or three years when the doctor acquires increased but supervised responsibility for patients and specialist skills;
3. *Higher specialist training* follows, lasting three to five years, and fits a doctor to be a consultant;
4. *Vocational training for general practice* is the statutorily prescribed three year training for NHS general practice (or its recognized equivalent);
5. *Independent practice* involves unsupervised responsibility for patients as a consultant, a principal in general practice or in independent private practice;
6. *Continuing medical education* is the continuing process whereby a doctor seeks to maintain her or his competence as an independent practitioner.

The attributes of the independent practitioners were outlined: the ability to solve clinical and other problems in medical practice; possession of adequate knowledge and understanding of the general structure and function of the human body and workings of the mind, in health and disease, of their interaction and of the interaction between man (*sic*) and his physical and social environment; possession of consultation skills; acquisition of a high standard of knowledge and skills in the doctor's specialty; willingness and ability to deal with common medical emergencies and other illnesses in an emergency; the ability to contribute appropriately to the prevention of illness and the promotion of health; the ability to recognize and analyse ethical problems so as to enable patients, their families, society and the doctor to have proper regard to such problems in reaching decisions; the maintenance of attitudes and conduct appropriate to a high level of professional practice; mastery of skills required to work within a team and, where appropriate, assume the responsibilities of team leader; acquisition of experience in administration and planning; recognition of the opportunities and acceptance of the duty to contribute, when possible, to the advancement of medical knowledge and skill; recognition of the obligation to teach others, particularly doctors in training.

Turning to the content of training, and emphasizing that the Council had no intention of duplicating the specialist guidelines already in existence, the recommendations first referred specifically to the inclusion in specialist training of content common to training in all specialties, including communication skills, practical skills, prevention of illness and promotion of health, teamwork, management, problem solving, knowledge and skills which cross specialty boundaries. Then followed the maintenance of high standards of practice, including: audit; the importance of teaching; the relevance of research to training in all specialties; and, finally, clinical academic medicine.

The third main section addressed the process of training, dealing with: the needs of the trainee and the responsibilities of the educational supervisor; the need for breadth and flexibility in training programmes; assessing the trainee; the criteria for approval of training posts; the duration of training; part-time training and job-sharing; career guidance.

The fourth section, acknowledging that the NHS supplies most of the funding, sets out the respective roles and responsibilities of the interested bodies—the GMC education committee, royal colleges, faculties and joint higher training committees, the national and regional levels. Three final sections deal with overseas qualifications, EC requirements and continuing medical education respectively.

Consistent with their usual pattern, in 1988 the Council and the education committee called a conference to discuss postgraduate training. One's impression from reports is that, despite the wide consultation, not everyone was happy. Sir Robert Kilpatrick, briefly chairperson of the education committee before becoming president, said in the annual report:

> The committee appreciates, of course, that time will be required before the recommendations may be fully implemented and therefore proposes to resume consideration of the matter in due course.
>
> Kilpatrick (1989b), p. 4

Within their documents on postgraduate education the education committee had recognized many of the problems which in the end were likely to require structural changes for their solution, but neither it nor Council had recommended any such changes. Probably two reasons explain this. First, there was a wish to establish a pattern of working relations with the royal colleges and others before recommending anything very drastic—the requirement imposed by regulation by professional consensus. Second, the Council was nervous throughout the 1980s of proposing legislation; the political atmosphere was not favourable to professionals in general and to medicine in particular, suggesting that there might be above-average hazards in requesting legislation—better to hope the dogs would snooze if not disturbed; clearly they were not very sound asleep.

So, despite all the talk and paper spent, by the end of the 1980s there had been no very radical change in the pre-registration year, nor in the content of undergraduate medical education. Apart from the addition of health centres—an important change—the only major change had been in the issue of new regulations as to the combination of training periods which could be taken. It had always been possible to divide the year into three four-month periods, so long as six months was in an aspect of medicine and six months in an aspect of surgery. In 1979 this had been made mandatory by regulation.

However, the start of a new era in the regulation of medical education had been signalled with a good deal of thinking, paper and consultation. The Council was aware that the education committee would not be able to make its wishes stick without a register of specialist qualifications. However, as we saw, all that had been achieved on this front by the start of the 1990s was the permission to include authorized specialist qualifications in the register.

From 1988 the education committee had begun a review of undergraduate medical education, preliminary to its decennial revision of its guidance, determined to tackle the overcrowding of the undergraduate curriculum (Kilpatrick, 1989, p. 6). The new chairperson, Professor David Shaw, in his 1989 report pointed out that the 1980 guidance had encouraged liberation of the curriculum but

> the shackles have not been loosened in any significant way. Ten years on, we have embarked on a further review, seeking to tackle the problems afresh.

Referring to the many obstacles in the way of reform, including those from teachers of old and new subjects, he added:

> Furthermore, under existing arrangements the newly fledged pre-registration house officer is often expected to take on clinical duties with more responsibility, and less supervision, than could possibly be consistent with our recommendations on general clinical training.
>
> Shaw (1989), p. 17

Tail-piece: the government 1991 white paper, the NHS and medical education

The proper clinical training of medical students and young doctors depends not only on their adequate educational supervision, but also on the availability of adequate posts. Here the interface with the NHS authorities and the Department of Health is crucial. From 1982 onwards the education committee had been concerned about the effects of public expenditure cuts on medical education. The first concerns were about university teaching and later increasingly about the effects of cuts in the NHS on clinical training. In 1986 the education committee for the first time found it necessary to exercise the 'concerned role' which Merrison had suggested for it in regard to resources. The committee formally conveyed to government its concern that standards of medical education were already compromised by lack of resource. It reported its concern at length to the profession in the *GMC Annual Report for 1986* (pp. 29–31).

Throughout the period we have been discussing there had been unrest among junior hospital doctors (JHDs). Dissatisfaction with the low pay and the long hours of continuous duty expected from them had led at the end of the 1970s to agreement that JHDs could claim overtime pay. The new conditions of hospital work and the continued hierarchical structure, with large differences in pay between top and bottom, had made a move of that kind inevitable. Senior doctors, among them Sir Robert Wright, indicated to me that the necessity for this agreement was a sad day for professionalism, which formerly had implied that a doctor in return for appropriate remuneration did whatever was required of her or him. The relative exploitation of JHDs was no new matter, however.

Discontent continued and became marked at the end of the 1980s and the beginning of the 1990s, as the NHS became more and more underfunded and doctors, along with all other NHS staff, had to deal with the trauma of yet another NHS reorganization—this one more radical than anything that had gone before. In October 1990 the BMA junior hospital doctors' committee initiated a survey of JHDs as to their willingness to undertake industrial action in pursuit of their claims. In January 1991 the Court of Appeal gave permission to a Dr Johnstone to proceed with his claim against the Bloomsbury Health Authority that they, his employer, had required unlawful amounts of overtime (*The Independent*, 11 January 1991).

Concerned with the 'eccentric and idiosyncratic' structure of post-graduate medical education, Kenneth Clarke, then Secretary of State for Health, issued a white paper in January 1991 proposing widespread reforms of postgraduate medical and dental education, including, for the first time, the earmarking of an education budget. This will be administered by 28 regional postgraduate deans, no longer appointed by universities alone; universities in conjunction with health authorities will employ the deans and administer the budget. Junior doctors hope that this may provide them with a consistent course structure and access to study leave they at present lack. At the time of writing the relationship of the GMC to these new arrangements is unclear. They remain statutorily responsible for the standards of postgraduate education up to full registration and for co-ordinating all education thereafter.

10

Registration and Education II: Overseas-qualified Doctors

The overseas committee

I can speak with less assurance about the overseas committee than I could about the education committee, not only because I was a member of the latter and never of the former, but also because the education committee publishes minutes of all its meetings as well as an annual report to Council. The overseas committee only publishes minutes about cases which have come before it for adjudication (see Chapter 12 for such disciplinary matters); no minutes of its other meetings are published, although a report is made to Council and printed. (This is also true of the registration committee.) While on the GMC, I was, of course, a party to the discussions in Council about the reports of the overseas and registration committees as well as those from the education committee. However, I have talked to other Council members about the committees I was not on, particularly about the overseas committee.

Responsibiity for establishing the sufficiency of the education received by doctors qualifying overseas rests not with the education committee, but with the overseas committee of the Council. Council deals with overseas-qualified doctors differently and separately from those qualified in the UK. Whereas in regulating UK-qualified doctors responsibility as to fitness to practise is divided between education, registration, conduct and health committees, where doctors qualified abroad are concerned until 1990 one overseas committee and its subcommittees dealt with all aspects: appropriateness of education, registration, discipline and conduct. In the case of those qualified overseas, the Council has defined all this work as coming under the general heading of registration, and the question of the suitability of such persons for registration is felt to have special features and is therefore dealt with separately. The education committee only becomes involved where UK institutions are concerned, as when, for example, after 1975 non-university examining bodies in the UK continued to admit direct to their final examinations graduates of universities abroad from which the Council had withdrawn recognition.

The Council had appointed a special committee in 1971 to examine the arrangements for registering the overseas-qualified doctors on which the health service had come to rely so heavily in the 1960s (see Chapter 5). Great unhappiness had been expressed by the medical profession, the health service and the overseas doctors themselves about these arrangements. The GMC had been accused of registering doctors who were not appropriately qualified and also of failing to register others who were so qualified. In 1972 the standing overseas committee was set up. When the special committee had completed the preparation of evidence on overseas doctors' registration for the Merrison committee it ceased to function, leaving the field to the standing committee.

The activities of the overseas committee involve the question whether, in general, the medical education offered by a university abroad guarantees the suitability of its graduates to practise medicine in the UK. If so, that university can be recognized by the GMC and its graduates accepted for full registration. This is essentially similar to the decision the education committee makes as to the sufficiency of UK university education. Originally recognition of universities abroad was a matter for the whole Council, as was UK medical education before 1970.

Since 1990 three committees deal with the matters which formerly were dealt with by its two subcommittees: F and L. Broadly speaking, subcommittee F (now overseas committee F) deals with questions to do with overseas doctors and full registration while subcommittee (now overseas committee) L deals with limited registration. Committee L began life as subcommittee T (for temporary), being renamed when 'temporary' registration was changed to 'limited'. At the outset in 1974 a subcommittee had been established to deal with matters concerning the conduct or character of applicants for limited registration (under Chapter XVI of the Standing Orders) rather than such questions being dealt with by the established disciplinary procedures of the Council (*GMC Minutes, CXI*, 1974, pp. 216–8; discipline is dealt with in detail in the following two chapters). The subcommittee also had power to deal with any other matters which the committee wished to delegate.

In 1975 the subcommittee's principal work was to establish weekly (mostly by post) whether overseas applicants for full registration had sufficient professional experience—this needed to be equivalent to the pre-registration year. However, the overseas committee's work would increase in 1976 by the decision that no doctor should have temporary registration unless she or he had the equivalent experience to that of the pre-reg. year; also the committee needed to consider individual cases of exemption from the TRAB tests. So a second subcommittee was set up and 'T' came into being—the original committee becoming F (for full). The work of the committees have changed somewhat over the years; for example, subcommittee L considers applications from universities overseas for acceptance of their qualifications for limited registration and F considers applicants for upgrading from limited to full registration which are not so routine that they can be dealt with in the office.

Composition of the overseas committee

To enable the extra work to be discharged and these two committees set up, the composition of the overseas committee was changed somewhat in 1975 both to enlarge it and to model it on the structure of the education committee rather than, as it initially was, on the executive committee. The overseas committee is elected annually by Council along with all the other standing committees. Initially it had 13 or 14 elected members and others co-opted. In 1976 there were 14 elected by Council (five elected members, four university representatives, three from the royal colleges, one medical Crown nominee and one lay member). In addition three further members were co-opted, all professors. As noted above, before 1979 there were no overseas doctors on the Council; none were brought in as advisers to the committee, although inviting non-members to attend some committee meetings as advisers was a common practice.

After 1979, two of the newly elected overseas doctors were elected by Council to serve on the overseas committee and a further one was co-opted. The committee was also increased in size: 19 members elected by Council (six each from the elected members, the university representatives and the royal colleges and one lay member). The president had always been an *ex officio* member of the committee so, with the co-opted members, the committee now totalled 23 when all the places were filled.

A review board was set up under the 1978 Medical Act to consider appeals against decisions of Council about the registration of doctors qualified overseas. The chairman and deputy chairman of this board were appointed by the president on the recommendations of the councils for postgraduate medical education and are not members of the Council. In addition the Council elected seven other members, one of whom must be overseas qualified. In 1979 a second overseas-qualified practitioner was also elected by the Council. The review board advises the president, who makes the final decision.

Establishing qualifications for entry

Temporary registration

Temporary registration had been introduced in 1947; tests to establish whether a doctor was qualified to be temporarily registered were decided on in 1973. In 1949 there had been less than 80 periods of temporary registration granted, and in 1953, there were 498. By 1963 the number had climbed to 2595. In 1974, when the Temporary Registration Assessment Board (TRAB) was established, 13,777 periods of temporary registration were granted involving 6897 doctors. The conditions for temporary registration were such that each certificate related to a post, so that the same doctor might well need more than one certificate a year.

The Board, chaired by Dr T. C. Hunt, was independent of the Council and included educational and linguistic experts. Linguistic and professional competence was to be tested. Initially the assessment was based on: a comprehension test of spoken English; a multiple choice question paper to test factual professional knowledge, covering medicine, surgery and obstetrics; a 'modified essay question' to test written professional English; and a *viva voce* examination to test practical professional knowledge as well as proficiency in English. Until very recently it was necessary for candidates to pass in all the components of the examination at the same sitting. Many doctors took the tests again and again, never managing to pass all components at once. So many doctors were taking the test four or more times that Council decided that from 1981 if a doctor failed the test severely after three attempts she or he would not be allowed to try again.

At first it was not thought possible (although it would be desirable) to include a clinical component. Simulations of clinical situations were added later. The tests were in a continual state of evolution throughout the first decade of their use. In 1985 a 'projected material examination' was introduced to test clinical aspects and in 1987 the 'medical short answer' paper was replaced by a different written examination involving clinical problem solving. The two together were thought to 'go a considerable way towards' an alternative to a full clinical examination, which remained impracticable on logistic and financial grounds (*GMC Annual Report for 1987*, p. 34). A new and more modern English comprehension test was introduced in 1988.

The 1978 Medical Act replaced temporary registration by limited registration. At the same time TRAB was replaced by PLAB (Professional and Linguistic Assessment Board), effectively simply making statutory the on-going arrangements. Table 10.1 shows the numbers of candidates and the numbers and proportions passing. There are, given the resits, more candidates than there are doctors involved.

Table 10.1 Clinical and linguistic tests: candidates and results 1975–1988

	TRAB Tests				PLAB Tests									
	1975[a]	1976	1977	1978	1979	1980	1981	1982	1983	1984	1985	1986	1987	1988[b]
Candidates	1019	1516	1663	1828	2420	2710	2978	2572	2259	2175	1984	1876	1734	1187[c]
Passes	352	510	532	770	919	1160	1208	954	742	554	418	428	435	383[c]
Per cent pass	34	34	32	37	38	43	41	37	33	25	22	23	25	32[c]

[a] 1975 figures are for the first nine months of operation of TRAB. All subsequent figures are for January to December of each year unless otherwise stated.
[b] Data have not yet been published for the years after 1988.
[c] Figures available only for the eight months January to August 1988 (General Medical Council, 1988a, p. 361); the overall pass rate for the year was reported at 30% (General Medical Council, 1988).

Sources: *GMC Minutes*; *GMC Annual Reports*.

What is perhaps most striking about this table is the low pass rate (around about a third) throughout the period and particularly how low it fell in 1986 and 1987. I shall return to this later.

Table 10.2 shows that there were always at least 50 and sometimes over 60 countries whose nationals sat the TRAB or PLAB tests. It also shows, from the time the TRAB tests started, the countries from which the three largest numbers of candidatures came, their pass rates and the average pass rate for each year. India is always there, Egypt almost always, Iraq until 1980, after which Pakistan and Sri Lanka appear. Of these three, Iraqi candidates have consistently above-average pass rates and Egyptians consistently below. Nigeria is noticeable as another country which, while never appearing in the top three, frequently in the late 1970s and early 1980s provided over 100 candidatures.

Full registration

Throughout the 1970s the process of withdrawing recognition from universities overseas proceeded. Ninety had been recognized in 1970; by 1976 only 23 were left. This severely restricted the number of overseas medical graduates entitled to full registration. A further restriction was introduced by the 1978 Medical Act whereby language proficiency had to be established before full registration could be granted.

Reciprocity, whereby there was mutual recognition of medical qualifications between the UK and other countries (a legacy of empire), came to an end in 1980 as signalled by the 1978 Act. Not all countries overseas had wished to maintain reciprocity. Alberta, Newfoundland and Nova Scotia pulled out in the 1970s; New Brunswick, Ontario and Quebec had already done so in the 1920s. From 1980, the individual recognition by the Council of the qualifications of specific universities was now the only direct route to full registration. By 1982 the number recognized had fallen to 21 to rise to 22 in 1984. From 1981 universities wishing to maintain their recognition were required to make annual returns.

From 1979 there were four routes to full registration. The first, just discussed, was to hold a recognized qualification. The second was to move from limited to full registration which could be done after a specified period of residence and an appropriate record. The third was for the doctor to requalify in UK. The fourth falls into another category: the temporary granting of full registration to a limited number of visiting specialists. Table 10.3 shows the numbers in each of these four categories from 1974; it also shows the number on the temporary or limited register for those years.

Table 10.2 TRAB and PLAB tests: candidates, countries and passes from 1975. Three countries with most numerous entries each year

	Countries	Candidates	Passes	% Pass	% Pass overall	Total countries
1975	India	236	100	42		
	Egypt	215	46	21		
	Iraq	103	49	47	34	52
1976	India	376	142	38		
	Egypt	315	88	28		
	Iraq	254	105	41	34	50
1977	India	421	142	34		
	Egypt	389	107	27		
	Iraq	246	109	44	32	52
1978	Egypt	411	147	36		
	India	405	150	37		
	Iraq	346	177	51	37	52
1979	India	631	225	36		
	Egypt	456	128	28		
	Iraq	328	137	42	38	58
1980	India	791	341	44		
	Egypt	433	137	34		
	Iraq	360	166	46	43	64
1981	India	946	407	43		
	Pakistan	411	147	36		
	Sri Lanka	368	234	64	41	62
1982	India	967	362	37		
	Pakistan	345	124	36		
	Sri Lanka	260	146	56	37	54
1983	India	957	348	36		
	Pakistan	344	117	34		
	Egypt	221	45	20	33	61
1984	–	–	–	–	25	–
1985	India	757	195	26		
	Pakistan	332	68	26		
	Egypt	203	20	10	22	60
1986	India	712	199	28		
	Pakistan	350	72	21		
	Egypt	169	23	14	23	56
1987	India	678	197	29		
	Pakistan	384	104	27		
	Egypt	144	28	20	25	57
1988	–	–	–	–	30	–

– Indicates data not available; no data have yet been published since 1988.

Sources: GMC annual reports, GMC minutes.

Table 10.3 Registration of overseas-qualified doctors

	1974	1975	1976	1977	1978	1979	1980	1981	1982	1983	1984	1985	1986	1987	1988	1989
Full registration granted to:																
Doctors holding recognized quals						1426	2990	1027	774	867	929	967	921	990	1010	1395
limited reg'n						227	657	342	271	360	574	737	620	785	623	682
requalified in UK						82	83	93	78	101	154	139	123	95	98	80
Visiting o'seas drs						30	41	35	42	41	39	26	43	45	22	26
Total full reg'n grants	1930	2741	3133	2800	2669[a]	1814	3771	1497	1165	1369	1696	1869	1707	1915	1753	2183
Limited reg'n granted to drs whose quals GMC accepts[a]																
Overall number	2391	1934	1021	–	–	6317	6206	5533	–	5641	5434	5241	5077	4815	4986	5546
Initial grants				1124	1365	1399	1682	1671	1473	1129	1123	1024	1034	1161	1433	1784
Total no. on limited reg'r[a, b]	–	–	6912	6555	5982	4339	5544	5308	5707	5938	5582	5085	4586	3876	3663	–

[a] Temporary registration until 14 February 1979 when limited registration began.
[b] Figures on the register are as at 1 January annually.

Source: GMC Annual Reports.

Clinical attachment and sponsorship

In 1966 the DHSS had established on a voluntary basis a scheme whereby overseas doctors could gain, through being attached to a consultant, experience of British hospital practice before taking up a post. From 1969 all overseas doctors were required to undertake such an attachment before taking up an NHS appointment and the Department authorized the payment of an allowance to them. In 1974 the GMC recognized that this process was not working well and tried to get it improved and linked to the TRAB test. The DHSS were unwilling to support the proposals without the support of the Joint Consultants Committee (JCC) which was not forthcoming. The scheme continued uneasily alongside the developing GMC arrangements. In 1979 the DHSS decided to abandon the scheme, telling the Council that of 1500 doctors who had undertaken mandatory clinical attachments after first passing the TRAB test, only one had been unsuccessful. TRAB's view was that for doctors who had passed their tests there was no need for the scheme. The GMC accepted the abandonment of what they had long felt was an unsatisfactory arrangement (*GMC Minutes*, 1974, pp. 224–230; 1976, pp. 310–311; 1980, pp. 326–327).

There was also a sponsorship scheme in existence whereby overseas doctors were, by prior arrangement, accepted to a training post under the tutelage of a consultant or similar senior doctor in the UK who had undertaken to provide and supervise their training. Such doctors were granted limited registration. Reviewing the situation in 1980, overseas subcommittee L concluded:

In general overseas qualified doctors in this category were carefully selected, well supervised and received satisfactory training in the posts and programmes arranged for them.

This contrasted in the subcommittee's view with the training and supervision accorded to many who had passed the PLAB test:

Many unsponsored ... arrived in the United Kingdom expecting to take up hospital posts under limited registration only to find they had difficulty in passing the PLAB test. Even when they did pass, they were more likely than not to obtain employment in a succession of service posts instead of being able to obtain a planned course of postgraduate training and experience in the specialty of their preference.

GMC Minutes, CXVIII (1981), p. 223

From then on the GMC, in conjunction with other bodies, national and international, decided to develop the sponsorship scheme. By 1987 the overseas committee was able to report that:

> During recent years the proportion granted [limited registration] after a PLAB test has fallen and sponsorship has become of greater importance, a valuable development in that suitable training posts are more likely to be obtained.
>
> *GMC Annual Report for 1987*, pp. 29–30

I have seen no systematic assessment of how well the scheme is thought to be working.

Further immigration controls

In the 1960s and 1970s the NHS had great need of doctors qualified overseas. There was concern to control the quality but not to staunch the supply. By 1980 the tide was turning: the products of the new British universities were coming on the market. The words 'medical unemployment' began to be uttered in the GMC corridors, for the first time, I would guess, since before the Second World War. Technically the GMC has nothing to do with manpower; in practice its actions greatly affect the supply of registered practitioners. The profession as a whole began to view the influx of overseas doctors in a different light.

The tone of Council activities to restrict and control immigrant doctors gets tougher and tougher at the beginning of the 1980s until the overseas committee feels it has the situation under control, when utterances become more beneficent. This did not really happen until the immigration rules were changed in 1985 to restrict doctors to a four-year permit-free stay in the UK. The 1978 Act had prevented the Council from granting limited registration for more than five years, although in chronological time that could be extended by doctors temporarily unemployed de-registering, so that those weeks or months did not count towards their total residence in the UK. About 100 did this in 1982. The *GMC Annual Report for 1982* advised those doctors who had not got full registration within the five years to go home (p. 35). I recall the anxiety this raised among the overseas doctors who wished the provisions of the Act relaxed. The effect of the 1985 rules was to prevent the full use of the five years which the 1978 Medical Act allowed. My information is that, given the overseas representation on the Council, the white British senior doctors had not been able to get the Council to agree to further restrictions and so had 'gone to government'— hence the rule change.

Table 10.1 shows that, starting low at 34% in 1975, rising to 43%, the pass rate for the TRAB/PLAB tests began to fall in 1981 and increasingly rapidly from 1983 to an all-time low in 1985, to rise again to 32% in 1988. This is noted by the GMC, but not analysed. How much may be attributed to the standard of the candidates and how much to a conscious or unconscious variation in the standards required to pass at a time of increasing restrictiveness, I cannot say.

Racial discrimination

Just as I was leaving the Council anxiety began to be expressed both outside and inside the Council about the appropriateness of recognizing for full registration medical schools in South Africa which practised apartheid. Technically their medicine might be excellent and conforming to UK standards, but what of the ethics the students learned about the administration of medicine?

In October 1984 a working party was set up to look at a number of problems relating to the grant of full registration to overseas-qualified doctors. In addition to Mr Innes Williams, the overseas committee chairperson, who also chaired the subcommittee, the working party consisted of nine people of whom one was lay (Dame Catherine Hall, a nurse) and one was an overseas doctor. In January 1985 a further overseas doctor was appointed and when one British professor's term of office ceased in February he was not replaced (thus for a month the committee had ten members).

Among the matters the committee considered was the allegation that

the recognition of overseas primary qualifications for the purpose of full registration was a relic of the imperial past irrelevant to current needs.

In response to which:

The working party agreed that there is an historical background to many of the Council's arrangements, but that this alone did not justify their revision.
GMC Minutes, CXXII (1985), p. 261

With regard to another allegation that

the teaching at some universities, although of requisite academic standard, might not adequately prepare graduates for practice in the United Kingdom where cultural relationships between doctor and patient or between doctors of one race and those of another might be quite different from those of the country of origin the working party

> were not aware of any complaints arising.
>
> *GMC Minutes* (1985), p. 262

The specific issue of South African universities was dealt with by reference to the law, counsel's opinion being sought on more than one occasion. This finally indicated that, under section 19 of the 1983 Medical Act,

> criteria applied by a medical school in relation to the admission of students could not in itself provide a sufficient justification for withdrawing recognition of the primary medical qualification.

Furthermore, registration could only be withheld from a person with a recognized qualification on grounds of the unfitness of that particular person (*GMC Minutes*, 1985, p. 290).

This whole episode has been referred to by senior GMC members involved as 'that fuss'—something which had to be overcome, contained, was a nuisance and which proved quite difficult. I gained no sense in interview that the opportunity had been taken of achieving greater understanding of the problems of race relations in the medical profession, about which see Anwar and Ali (1987).

Establishing qualifications for entry: EC-qualified doctors

The situation with regard to EC-qualified doctors is greatly different from that of those qualified overseas. All that is required of the GMC so far as EC doctors are concerned is to establish that they are nationals of a member State and that they hold recognized medical qualifications from a member state. Doctors may hold the qualifications of one country and be nationals of another.

The free movement of doctors throughout the EC began in December 1976, although the Order in Council was not made until 11 May 1977 to be effective on 10 June. This Order specified that doctors entering from Europe would have to take a language test after six months (Draper, 1978). Given the imposition of language tests on overseas-qualified doctors, the GMC had been most anxious that this provision should be made. However, the provision gave rise at once to much continental criticism, the upshot of which was that the UK government found they had to give in. The language test consequently ceased on 1 August 1981, much to the distress of the GMC's executive committee, upset at this reminder of their reduced sovereignty as to who should be registered to practise in the UK, but also because of the imbalance with overseas doctors and the hazards for patients. However, from 1 August it became the responsibility of NHS employing authorities and family practitioner committees

> to satisfy themselves that an EEC doctor seeking to work here could communicate effectively in English.
>
> *GMC Annual Report for 1981*, p. 9

It was arranged that EC doctors could take the PLAB test.

It had been noted in the *Annual Report for 1979* that 60 candidates in the PLAB test were EC doctors of whom 49 passed. However, between 1 August 1981 and 31 December 1987 only three EC doctors took the test. The GMC decided to look further into how health authorities were assuring themselves about language. The registrar wrote to the DHSS in 1982 and again in 1983. Thereafter the matter was not referred to either in the *Minutes* or the *Annual Reports* of the Council.

Few EC doctors claimed registration at first, but the number gradually grew in the 1980s, more than doubling between 1986 and 1987, as Table 10.4 shows. Most registrations have come from Germany, followed by Greece, but many countries are represented, as Table 10.5 shows. That table also distinguishes the countries where the doctors qualified and their nationalities.

The increasing movement of European doctors and their assimilation to full registration without GMC intervention contrasts starkly with the situation of other overseas-qualified doctors. The arrangements for their regulation remain distinct and were much more tightly controlled by the 1990s

Table 10.4 Fully registered EC-qualified practitioners

	No. added each year	Total fully registered[a]
1977	85	85
1978	109	194
1979	124	318
1980	134	452
1981	184	636
1982	264	900
1983	327	1227
1984	302	1529
1985	332	1861
1986	445	2306
1987	995	3301
1988	1309	4610

[a] A cumulative total from which some will have removed their names (numbers unknown).

Source: *GMC Minutes, CXXVI* (1989), pp. 36–37.

Table 10.5 EC-qualified doctors granted full registration from 10 June 1977 to 31 December 1988

	Countries where qualifications granted	Countries of nationality
Belgium	301	281
Denmark	83	80
France	189	174
Germany	1029	992
Greece	851	868
Ireland[a]	659	608
Italy	690	631
Luxembourg	0	7
Netherlands	549	551
Portugal	46	45
Spain	213	208
UK	0	165
Total	4601	4601

[a] Until 30 April 1985 doctors qualified in the Republic of Ireland were registered in the UK on the same basis as UK-qualified doctors. These are not included in the statistics on Ireland.

Source: *GMC Annual Reports.*

than they had been earlier. In addition to the special status accorded them, overseas doctors were also caught up, as were their UK colleagues, in all the problems of postgraduate education and the tensions between service and education in the junior years which were discussed in the previous chapter.

11

Maintaining a Register of the Competent I: Discipline and Health

The maintenance of a register of the competent is fundamental to the regulation of a profession.

Merrison Report (1975), paragraph 1

Having ensured in the ways it has chosen that those on the registers are competent to practise, the second duty of the GMC is, as Merrison points out, to remove those who are incompetent. The GMC has a control mechanism for this purpose which now bifurcates into two: the professional conduct committee and the health committee. It is currently considering a third: some system with local bases nationwide to assess rather than control the performance of practitioner. Until the 1978 Act, however, there was only one type of discipline available to Council. So that doctors may know what is expected of them, a committee on standards of professional conduct and on medical ethics (known as the standards committee for short) has since 1963 prepared guidelines as to proper professional practice, *Professional Conduct and Discipline: Fitness to Practise*, known as the blue pamphlet or the blue book. This superseded earlier and briefer *Notices* (*GMC Annual Report for 1981*, p. 18).

Discipline until 1973

Initially, the whole Council dealt with matters of discipline. Not until the 1950 Medical Act which followed the 1944 Goodenough Report was a separate disciplinary committee set up, a change not popular with the Council (Draper, 1983). Table 11.1 shows that the work of the committee was small then in comparison with that of the present day. To some extent the increase in the number of registered medical practitioners explains the increase in the number of cases. This is not the whole story, however.

Table 11.1 Meetings of the disciplinary and professional conduct committees: 1955–1988

Years	Average no. mtgs per yr	Average no. days met per year
1955–1961	2.3	5.9
1962–1973	3.5	16
1974–1979	3.7	21
1980	Disc 5	Disc 10
	PCC 2	PCC 5
1981	Disc 3	Disc 3
	PCC 6	PCC 23
1982–1988	8.3	43.5

Sources: From 1955 to 1974 inclusive. Tabulations, *1974 Minutes of the General Medical Council Vol. CX1*, GMC, 1974, pp. xix,xx.

From 1975 to 1978 inclusive, Tabulations, *1978 Minutes of the General Medical Council, Vol. CXV*, GMC, 1978, pp. xx,xxi.

From 1979 onwards by extrapolation of the minutes of the disciplinary and professional conduct committees, *Minutes of the General Medical Council, Vols CXVI–CXXV*, GMC, 1978–1988.

Note: Until and including 1979 data refer to the disciplinary committee; during 1980 and 1981 both the disciplinary committee (Disc) and the professional conduct committee (PCC) sat; these years are consequently shown separately: for 1982 and subsequently the data refer to the professional conduct committee.

Lord Cohen of Birkenhead took over as president in November 1961. The first increase, the doubling of the number of days on which the committee met, from six in 1961 to 12 in 1962, may be attributed to the more active style of presidency which he instituted compared with that of his predecessor Sir David Campbell who had held office for 12 years from 1949 (Martin Draper, personal communication).

However, in Lord Cohen's day the physical arrangements for sittings of the disciplinary committee remained much the same as they had been when Sir David Campbell was president:

> The scene in mind is that of the large Council Chamber, tall and lengthy, with a bow-window on the western wall, one summer day when a doctor is appearing before the Disciplinary Committee to answer a charge (say) of adultery with a patient. The strong, hot sun of a May afternoon glows through the blue, gold and vermilion of the arms of the twelve Presidents in the stained-glass window, and fills with light the lofty Chamber, decorated in the late eighteenth century style. Busts or portraits of past presidents look down from the oak-panelled walls. The Public Gallery at one end of the Chamber is crowded. Facing the bow-window, the doctor sits in his 'dock', with counsel or solicitors representing the parties at a table in front of him, and beyond them the long dais under the window where the President, Legal Assessor, and Registrar are sitting. In the centre of the chamber, to right and left of the lawyers' table, the nineteen members of the committee occupy their desks.
>
> Pyke-Lees (1958)

At that time the whole disciplinary committee sat on all cases. What Pyke-Lees called the 'dock', in which the defendant doctor stood, was still used in 1971. A member new in that year, who then as now identified strongly with the defendant doctor, described it to me as a box raised above the floor, such that if the doctor stepped back unwarily she or he would have fallen 'down a pit'. The proceedings had the formality found in a court of law.

Changes in 1973

Sir John (now Lord) Richardson, when elected president in succession to Lord Cohen in November 1973, made a number of changes to reduce the formality of the proceedings. The mace which used to be ceremonially carried into Council meetings now never appears, to the regret of some, including the member who so much objected to the 'dock'. Nobody now sits on the dais during disciplinary hearings; all parties are on a level. But what was greater informality in 1973 itself now appears formal. The formality is induced by the relative positions of the parties round a table and the presence of legal representatives of both the Council and the defendant doctor (although none wear gowns or wigs) as well as by the chairperson's gavel.

My induction: an example of discipline in 1974

The first week was not untypical except that a number besides myself were new there had just been elections). We were called together at 10.15 a.m. for a briefing in camera. The chairperson explained the rules of procedure: the most important point was that so far as the evidence in a case was concerned, we had to be 'certain so we were sure' before we could decide that a charge had been found proved—the standards were those of a criminal court. In practice we found that we were reminded of this quite often either by the chairperson or by the legal assessor who always sat with us.

The disposal decisions

We were introduced to the cards of questions which guided the decision-making process. There were two kinds of cases: those where a doctor had been already convicted in the courts and those where there was a charge of serious professional misconduct (SPM for short—although I never heard that shortening used in the Council chamber). Where a doctor was before us because she or he had been convicted in a court of law, she or he usually admitted the conviction at the start of the proceedings. Where it was a conduct charge, a decision had first of all to be made as to whether the facts alleged in the charges were proved.

The standard of proof required was high. It was that of the criminal courts, i.e. the facts had to be proved beyond all reasonable doubt. Members might be sure in their own minds in the way in which all of us judge social events, but could not be sure beyond all reasonable doubt. It might be that some of the facts alleged were found proved to this standard and others not; in that case those parts of the charge would have to be dropped.

The admission of the conviction or the proof of the charges in SPM cases constituted the first stage of the hearing; in the second stage the committee had to decide how to dispose of the case. When a conviction had been admitted or SPM proved beyond reasonable doubt, the following choices were open to the disciplinary committee:

to conclude the case
to admonish and conclude the case, or
   suspend,
   suspend forthwith,
   erase,
   erase and suspend forthwith.

There was also an option of postponement.

The committee might find a doctor guilty of SPM or it might accept the findings of a conviction but then not find that this required serious punishment, either because of the nature of the offence or because the doctor had already been punished enough. In such a case the committee would decide that it was 'sufficient to conclude the case'. More often a doctor found guilty of SPM would be admonished. She or he was then read a homily and the admonishment would go on the doctor's record, which would conclude the case.

In worse cases the committee would have to decide whether to erase or suspend. This seemed to depend upon a mixture of the seriousness of the offence and the likelihood of rehabilitation.

Pleas in mitigation from supportive colleagues or patients would be heard at this stage. Suspension of registration would be for a period of a few months up to a year. Suspension 'forthwith', which meant that the doctor was from that moment unable to practise, would be ordered where it was thought that the doctor was a continuing danger to her or his patients. Otherwise suspension became operative after 28 days. This allowed the doctor time to organize matters but also to appeal. Appeal is to the Privy Council but only on the ground that the hearing had not been properly conducted. Suspension had been brought in to deal with cases of illness (see below).

Erasure was for offences which indicated the practitioner was a serious danger to public and profession. As with suspension erasure would take effect in 28 days unless immediate suspension was also decided upon. Applications for restoration could be made ten months later; whether it would be granted is something else again.

Postponement, that is postponement of the judgement, was most commonly used to give a doctor a chance to change her or his ways before a final decision was reached as to whether the doctor was guilty of SPM and should be admonished, suspended or erased. Before the setting up of the health committee, postponement was commonly used for the surveillance of doctors who were drug or alcohol abusers.

My first week's cases

On that first morning a hazy outline of all of this was as much as one could grasp. After our induction the proceedings began at 10.30 as they usually did, at least for the first day. The gavel was struck and the hearings began. There were nine cases heard that week. Six of them were resumed hearings, the remaining three being cases considered for the first time. The six cases were all cases of convictions and all involved the abuse of drugs, although one also involved a drunk driving charge.

The first called was a man whose case had already been twice postponed before, having been first heard eight months previously. He was MRCS Eng., LRCP Lond. 1947, MBBS 1947 Lond. His conviction in 1974 was for drunk driving and associated charges—he refused a breath test. Fined £100 and costs and disqualified from driving for 18 months, he had also had charges proved against him of acquiring controlled drugs for self-administration. His case was concluded and he was discharged, it being decided from documents received that he had made satisfactory progress.

The second case concerned two convictions in 1963 and 1973, involving failure to keep a register of dangerous drugs and wrongful possession of dangerous drugs; he had been fined £150 on the first and £200 on the second conviction. An MRCS Eng., LRCP Lond. 1944, he presented as a very sad person. His case had already been postponed three times, having first come before the committee more than two years previously. The doctor seemed to have made progress, but the committee was not satisfied and further referred the case, telling the doctor that he should continue psychiatric treatment and produce a psychiatrist's report before appearing again in 12 months time. This doctor never reappeared: he died the following February.

The third man to appear had qualified MB ChB 1938 Glasgow. His conviction in 1975 had also been to do with the wrongful purchase of controlled drugs and failing to keep a register; he had been fined £25. The committee concluded his case, implying that for the offence committed the court's punishment, along with having had to appear before the disciplinary committee, was sufficient. It seems he had collected his conviction because his estranged wife told on him.

The fourth case was a man who graduated from Glasgow MB ChB in 1954 and achieved his FRCS Edin. 1961. He had been convicted and fined £75 in 1975 for unlawfully possessing controlled drugs. His case had been postponed four months earlier. The evidence he produced satisfied the committee, which concluded his case. I was to see him more than once again, since he reappeared about a year later on a new but similar charge.

Then followed a man who appeared angry and anxious, and whose case had been postponed four months before. Qualified in 1954 MB BS Lond., he had been convicted in 1975 on several charges: obtaining drugs by deception, unlawful possession, failing to keep a register and unlawfully destroying drugs. He had been fined a total of £500 and £50 costs. Apparently he had not co-operated with his psychiatrist, and in the absence of satisfactory reports, the committee postponed his case for a further four months, calling for a psychiatrist's report to be available for that meeting.

The final resumed drug case was a woman, a sad waif and stray sort of person, who it was whispered had twice tried to commit suicide. She had qualified in 1960 LRCP Edin., LCRS Edin., LRFPS Glasgow, MB ChB Edin. She had been convicted of charges including obtaining drugs by deception and unlawfully possessing controlled drugs, fined £500 and had first come before the committee four months previously. Now the committee, judging she was not yet rehabilitated, postponed her case for 12 months, again calling for a psychiatrist's report and advising her to take treatment. She also was somebody I saw again but who died before any resolution was reached.

In all those cases the offences had occurred for self-administration. The doctors were not charged with improperly using their powers to prescribe controlled drugs to addicts. That morning's cases were all of 'sick doctors' who, after the implementation of the 1978 Act, would be referred to the health committee. The doctors, and certainly the last one, were thought to be more of a danger to themselves than to their patients. I got no flavour of what we really knew about their performance with patients. Indeed, one rarely did.

Lunch, preceded by a good array of preprandial drinks, consisted, as always, of excellent food well served by an outside caterer who regularly sent along the same women (known to all the doctors as 'girls', albeit one was a grandmother) to wait on us. A bell summoned us to the committee after lunch, as it had in the morning.

After lunch we heard a case of a man who apparently had never passed any examinations, but who had managed to get a certificate MRCS Eng. LRCP Lond. from the conjoint board in 1975. He was charged with offering false certificates in his application for Part II and also when applying for various jobs; in addition he had pretended to have held posts which he had never held. The problem with this case was that since he had never taken an exam he could not be a qualified medical practitioner; if he was not qualified how could we have jurisdiction over him? On the other hand he was on the medical register. Clearly he was not qualified to be on the register and it was necessary to get him off it. To this end, and despite the heart searchings, he was treated as if he were qualified. The charges were heard and the facts with minor amendment were found proved. This non-doctor was consequently found to be guilty of SPM and his registration was suspended forthwith. (I do not understand why he was not erased—a legal nicety I presume.)

I could not help finding this case very amusing but my medical colleagues took it very seriously indeed and were clearly not able to share a joke about it; they could not even take mild teasing in the lunch break. I noticed that the commissioner, the uniformed person—from the Peace Corps I think—who looks after everybody on these occasions, also found it funny. One could see the doctors' anxiety: the GMC's prime task is to keep a register of the qualified; to find they had registered an unqualified rogue challenged the whole competence of the Council. Undoubtedly it *is* a serious matter to have the untrained in practice (see the later section on *Paper Mask*).

The case that followed had been scheduled to be heard straight after lunch, but the counsel for the defence was delayed in court. Such rearrangements did not often happen, but the superiority of the law was acknowledged. The respondent, qualified MB ChB St Andrews 1947, had been convicted in 1976 on three charges of gross indecency (between November 1974 and August 1975). Pleading guilty, he had been sentenced to 18 months prison suspended for two years. He admitted the conviction. He was considered to be sick and seemed to accept that judgement. The committee referred him to a consultant psychiatrist and postponed the case for 12 months.

That ended our day's work; it was five to six—we had run over our 5.30 finishing time for the convenience of the respondent doctor's counsel. It suited us as well because it meant that we could start freshly in the morning on what was predicted to be the most difficult case of the week: we were warned that we might have to sit all week if not into the weekend.

In the morning we began the case of a doctor, a man, qualified MB BS 1966 Sind. There was no conviction: he was charged with writing prescriptions for controlled drugs otherwise than in the course of bona fide treatment—some of these for persons not on his NHS list and some for persons known to be addicted. In evidence it emerged he had charged £3 a time for these drugs (at 1975 prices), some written on NHS scripts. Two accounts of how his behaviour came to light circulated in the corridors: one that the pharmacist reported him; the other that two journalists visited the doctor posing as addicts and later exposed him in the *News of the World*. The journalists were important witnesses. Others were the mother of a, now dead, addict whom the respondent doctor had supplied and a probation officer whose work was being disrupted by the respondent doctor's prescribing habits which undermined the treatment other doctors were offering to addicts. Inevitably there was evidence from the drug squad. The defence counsel was unable to break down the prosecution witnesses, all of whom, including the mother of the dead addict, were clear, coherent and strong.

We rose at 5.30 p.m. to return again the next morning. Then for the first time I had the strange experience of coming back into the Council chamber to find the witness, the lawyers and the respondent doctor just where we had left them the night before. The odd feeling may have been strengthened in this case because we had stopped in the middle of the probation officer's evidence when it had become clear there was a good bit still to come. While I got used to this phenomenon in hearings which lasted several days, I never really got to the point of not noticing it; it was rather like returning to a TV drama after the commercials; it somehow added to the apparent unreality of the whole thing, or was it serving to remind one that there was another world out there?

When the doctor himself gave evidence, he appeared blustering and self-righteous; he had difficulty obeying the 'rules of the game'. He did nothing to help his case. His evidence ran over until the following day, Thursday. When the addresses by counsel were completed and we retreated into camera, the chairman having hit the table with his gavel and ordered 'Strangers will withdraw', we were quickly able to readmit them for the chairperson to announce we had found the facts proved and the doctor thereby guilty of SPM. Having announced this finding we once more retired into camera. Again 'strangers' were quickly readmitted to hear a verdict that the doctor should be erased from the register and suspended forthwith. The hearing had taken two and a half days and we did not after all have to stay into the weekend; it had been a sad tale of clumsily misused professional power.

That week's work did not entirely cover all the kinds of cases that one might hear and it was unusual in one respect. We erased one practitioner 'forthwith' and suspended another, the pretender, also 'forthwith'. Such sentences did not happen every week.

Cases which surprised me

I came to recognize cases and outcomes such as those I have described as what might be expected. There were, however, times when I was surprised. These I shall present as types of case and outcome, rather than reporting actual cases, because to understand what was going on reference has to be made to the way cases were handled *in camera*. None of these 'cases' actually exist in the GMC files: they are typifications only, about which readers may say 'she's talking about so-and-so'. She is not, but about a fiction like the typical 'so-and-so' whose case comes to the reader's mind.

Let us imagine, for example, a doctor, a man, who had failed to visit and treat some children. An attempt had been made in defence to put the blame on the mothers (who, incidentally, were very roughly handled by the defence counsel). The tough verdict that the respondent doctor was guilty of SPM prevailed because the senior doctors on the panel, and in particular the university doctors, took a strong line, saying among other things that it was the doctor's and not the mother's business to diagnose. However, although the facts were proved and the doctor found guilty of SPM, the conclusion was that the doctor should be admonished and the case concluded. This seemed to me to be pretty lenient for a doctor whose actions had put children's lives at risk. When I privately asked the chairperson in such types of case why that had been seen as a sufficient verdict, I was told 'because the doctor had already been punished enough', having already had a number of fines from the local practitioner committee, amounting to something like £300, in all and having had the case hanging over his head for three years. I guess this was an example of what members meant when they talked about the committee tempering justice with mercy.

In such cases the university doctors were tougher than those in daily practice. This did seem to happen quite often—those a bit detached from the daily fray tended to put the greater good of the profession over compassion for the particular practitioner. Later I tested statistically to see if that was always the case. The trend went in the expected direction but was not conclusive, not surprisingly given the small numbers and the many threads in any one case: divisions could easily develop between practitioners for other reasons than their position within the profession.

In another type of case, also a charge of failure to visit and treat, the use of the deputizing service was at issue. One committee member, a GP, suggested that it would be inappropriate to come down hard because of the widespread use of deputizing services; another GP was inclined to be tough because any misuse brought deputizing services into disrepute. Also involved in this case were issues to do with inappropriate delegation. Only one other member, a university professor of long standing, took a really serious view of the doctor's behaviour. In the end he and I were the only ones, after a finding of SPM had been reached with great difficulty, to vote for erasure. (As in a court of law, 'strangers' can guess when there is difficulty reaching a conclusion because of the length of the *in camera* session.) The *in camera* sessions on the finding of facts and on the appropriate punishment were long. My view was that leniency would condone SPM and this would not be good for the profession. The final decision was suspension, a disposal option brought in to help sick doctors but now also being used for penal offences.

My third imaginary case was where a great deal of evidence suggested that a doctor had not only failed to visit and treat but had written a prescription (on telephone information) that was lethal and caused the death of a person; and furthermore, that he had subsequently tried to destroy the evidence and influence the coroner. He was a man I felt might have been a friend of mine; he seemed a caring sort of GP. From a practitioner's point of view his was very much a case of I there but for the grace of God'—all were, but ones of this type more so than most; the mistake had been made when the doctor answered the phone while he was very busy in the surgery.

Proving the facts in a case like this was not easy: all those who initially voted 'hard' (including myself) were university professors. The final decision that the doctor was not guilty of SPM took two and a half hours to reach and was on a narrow vote. A case like that may have been a doctor's nightmare, but is also a patient's worst terror. Such decisions I found incredible.

The ethos of 1970s discipline

These accounts may give some of the flavour of GMC discipline in the mid-1970s. We spent our days, but not our nights, at the GMC when cases were being heard. It was not a total institution but it did have some encompassing qualities. The whole medical way of understanding the world and managing one's life within it was shared by all but the lay members present—and of course the paid officers, the legal assessors and stenographers. One became locked into the doctors' values, locked also into the arguments of the particular case and all its human qualities. I found I had to remind myself that a doctor now found guilty of SPM upon whom the verdict of 'suspension forthwith' had been passed had in all probability been continuing in practice ever since the charge had been laid. What had he been up to since then? Such questions have to be asked. In cases where there had been a conviction for a serious offence the relevant NHS authority had probably removed her or him from duty; but this could not apply to private practitioners. The law had imprisoned some. In any event it was not the GMC's disciplinary procedures which had first removed this public menace from the scene in which she or he might do damage.

There were other puzzling things. The majority of, but not all, doctors who came before the discipline committee were GPs. Did GPs really do more wrong things than hospital doctors? Was it, as the doctor members said, that in hospital colleagues are watching and a miscreant doctor will be pulled up, whereas in much general practice there are not those sorts of watchdogs? Or is it that in hospital there are colleagues who will cover up and witnesses from other professions are reluctant to come forward? Could it be that the *de facto* complaints procedure which the GP contract and the service committees offered was simply a more effective way of uncovering unprofessional behaviour than any of the hospital procedures? A different sort of study would be needed to answer such questions.

A great many who were charged with SPM were overseas doctors (not counting those applying for registration who appeared in another way; see the next chapter). Was this because they, being less familiar with the rules of British medical practice, broke them more often, or because of general failure to understand our ways of life? Was it because, being less familiar with the rules, they were less able to break them without being found out? Was it that there were not people to cover for them because they were not really members of the club, not quite in the fraternity, despite their full registration? Could it have been that, in the cases that were passed through for the full treatment meted out by the disciplinary committee, there was discrimination, most likely unconscious, for that is how much discrimination works?

Again I cannot say, but I do know that of the 34 new cases I sat on from 1976 to 1980, 17 had qualified overseas. Of the 120 doctors who appeared before the disciplinary panels in the same period (many reappearing for resumed hearings and some for new offences), 43 qualified overseas and 77 in the UK. A suggestion that there might be bias against overseas doctors in the examination of complaints had at one time been put to the president. He told me he had examined it and found it to be untrue; he gave no details. As noted above, were there such discrimination at work in any facet of the process, it would have been largely unconscious, based on stereotypes and assumptions rather than on any deliberate intention and might operate at any point from the initial reporting of the case to its reaching the disciplinary committee.

My research cannot answer the questions I have posed. All I can say is that I saw some pink-faced rogues and some brown-faced rogues as well as some of each who seemed to have been broken by life. But I remain uncomfortable about the high proportion of the non-white who were disciplined—uncomfortable because there may have been discrimination and also uncomfortable in the public interest at the thought that perhaps only a small proportion of unprofessional white doctors may have come before us. This raises the whole question of how cases came to be heard by the discipline committee.

How cases came to the Council

Cases reach the Council by a variety of routes. Where a doctor had been disciplined within the NHS it was the responsibility of the Department of Health to inform the GMC. Other officials might report a practitioner they were worried about. Members of the public may also complain of a practitioner's alleged misconduct. Unlike public officials, members of the public who wished to pursue a complaint had to support it by one or more statutory declarations, that is, statements declared in a prescribed form before a Commissioner for Oaths—rather a forbidding procedure.

The police or the Home Office are required to notify the Council of any registered medical practitioners who have been convicted in a criminal court. This includes everything from a drunk driving charge to cases involving the Home Office drug squad and those where a doctors' right to prescribe controlled drugs has been withdrawn. The Council on many occasions complained about long delays in notifications and made renewed attempts to get the matter improved. Quite apart from the problem that a doctor who was no longer fit might be continuing to practise, this also meant that, by the time of a hearing, the evidence was so old it was hard to assess whether there had been SPM.

Serious professional misconduct

The Council is only concerned if there has been SPM; it may regret other types of misdemeanour, but has no jurisdiction over them. What actually amounts to SPM? It was first termed 'infamous conduct in a professional respect', and Lord Justice Lopez in 1894 defined SPM thus:

> If a medical man [sic] in the pursuit of his profession has done something with regard to it which will be reasonably regarded as disgraceful or dishonourable by his brethren of good repute and competency, then it is open to the General Medical Council, if that be shown, to say that he has been guilty of infamous conduct in a professional sense.
>
> Quoted in GMC (1976)

In 1930 Lord Justice Scruton said:

> Infamous conduct in a professional respect means no more than serious misconduct according to the rules, written or unwritten, governing the profession.
>
> Quoted in GMC (1976)

Telling the profession what SPM is

As mentioned at the start of this chapter, the GMC publishes a 'blue book' to guide the profession as to what is proper conduct. Since 1979 the Council has been able to offer guidance beyond those areas where infringement is likely to lead to a charge of SPM (Richardson, 1980, p. 6). I analysed in some detail the changes which have taken place in the guidance between 1976 and 1987 (see Stacey, 1990). The blue pamphlet of 1976 was principally concerned with intra-professional ethics, the regulation of competition, for example, or the demeaning of colleagues. Little of the guidance related to the public interest, save in the important area of adultery, but significantly it was not only adultery with a patient, but any adultery, deriving one assumes, from the nineteenth century notions of 'gentlemanly behaviour'.

Taken overall, the blue book of 1987 is much different. Larger and more discursive, it still devotes a good deal of space to intra-professional ethics but contains more that is patient-oriented: for example about the confidentiality of the information which a doctor may have acquired about a patient, standards of medical care of patients, and an extensive section on relations with the pharmaceutical industry. A number of the more radical changes seem to have been a response to pressure from outside the Council, from the media, patients' associations and government. These will be dealt with more fully in the following chapter, where the Monopolies Commission's ruling about the permissibility of advertising will also be discussed. Suffice it to say here that the pressures often served to cause changes which a number of members already felt to be necessary.

What happened to complaints received?

The responsibility as to what should happen to a complaint received formally rests entirely with the president. Until Sir John (now Lord) Richardson's day, the president issued instructions to the office that they could act on certain types of complaint which were outside the Council's jurisdiction and looked at all other cases himself. Doing this and chairing the penal cases and disciplinary committees had attracted adverse comment. Lord Richardson consequently nominated a person, normally the chair of penal cases, to act as preliminary screener for him.

Before the 1978 Act the president had the following disposal routes available to him. He could conclude that SPM was not at issue and request the office to so inform the complainant. In the case of not-too-serious first offences he might send a letter of warning to the offending practitioner; cases which he inferred were potentially more serious, i.e. might amount to SPM, and convictions, he forwarded to the penal cases committee for preliminary investigation. Before, however, he forwarded a complaint of potential SPM he would have to decide not only whether, were the charge proved, it might be deemed to be SPM, but also 'whether the facts alleged were capable of proof' (Hill, 1975, p. 10).

In the 1970s this whole procedure was shrouded in a great deal of mystery. We know that in 1974 the 'Council received ... 847 complaints or letters about professional conduct from members of the public or of the profession' (Hill, 1975, p. 12). Of these, the penal cases committee received less than 100 (75 convictions, 22 possible SPMs); the disciplinary committee heard 39 cases (but involving charges under 46 heads) and we know that 22 others were dealt with by warning letters to the doctor.

Sir Denis Hill did not mention how many had been dealt with by the office, with the president's agreement, in a short note telling the complainants that their complaint fell outside the jurisdiction of the Council or referring them to the NHS procedures. This upset many complainants, who had not understood the relevance of the NHS complaints procedures or the niceties of what was defined as SPM; most of them would not have gone to the extent of complaining to the GMC were it not that they thought their grievance serious. Yet, on inquiring about the large gap between the number of complaints received and the number which were forwarded to

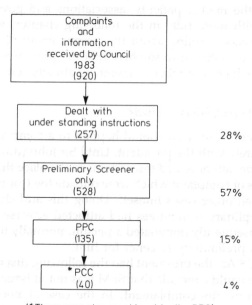

Figure 11.1 Complaints procedure 1983.
Source: *GMC Annual Report for 1983*, p. 21

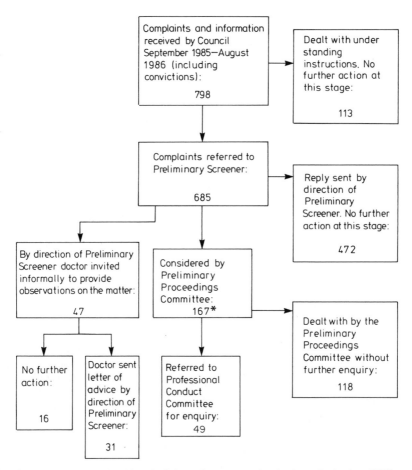

(*Includes one case in which the information was received prior to September, 1985)

Figure 11.2 Complaints procedure 1986.
Source: *GMC Annual Report for 1986*, p. 16

the disciplinary committee, one always received the assurance that 'most of them' came from deranged persons. 'If you saw them, Margaret, you would see that they were clearly deranged'; but one did not see them and I was never offered any examples to look at (I did not ask, either). However, my studies of complaints, complainers and complaining led me to be sceptical: no doubt a few were mad, but many more were seriously and rationally aggrieved. There are two issues here: what is legally considered to be SPM and how SPM was and is interpreted by the president and the relevant disciplinary committees of the Council.

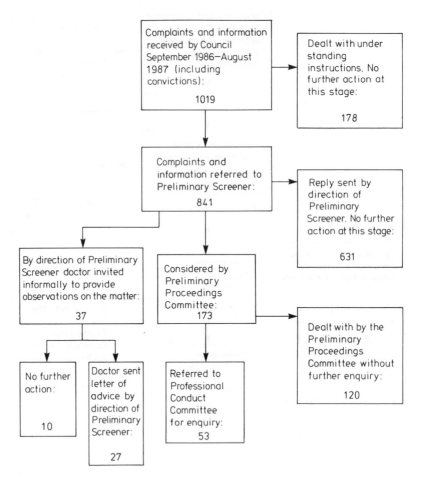

Figure 11.3 Complaints procedure 1987.
Source: *GMC Annual Report for 1987*, p. 17

Over the years rather more information has been made available about
what happens to complaints. In 1983 the flow diagram reproduced as
Figure 11.1 was published in the *Annual Report*. This deals only with conduct cases; unfitness to practise for health reasons was now dealt with
separately; I deal with that in a section below. It is unclear what relation
complaints about health bear to the total shown as 'complaints and
information received'.

The flow diagram showed public and practitioner how many cases were
dealt with under standing instructions (28%) how many by the preliminary
screener alone (57%) the proportion heard by the preliminary proceedings

committee (PPC) (15%) and the small number (4%) reaching the professional conduct committee (PCC). However since the number of complaints reported in that year is not comparable with the total of those handled it is unclear what the denominator is. The following year a similar flow diagram indicates similar proportions but makes no attempt to offer percentages.

In 1986 a somewhat more sophisticated flow diagram was produced (see Figure 11.2) giving greater detail of all the ways in which complaints were dealt with. It makes clearer how the preliminary screener disposes of cases without referral to the PPC and confirms that only a small proportion ever reach the PCC. In 1988 (see Figure 11.3) some further details are added (e.g. how the PPC disposed of cases) and some left out—we no longer know what the preliminary screener did about cases where he had invited the doctor to comment. The new-style 1989 *Annual Report* no longer gives a flow diagram.

The cases that are taken seriously

Those cases which reached the penal cases committee, or nowadays the PPC, and were passed from there to the discipline committee (now PCC) could be said to be the most serious. Table 11.2, showing the cases heard in 1974 when Denis Hill discussed discipline, gives an indication of the way in which the GMC lists cases.

While it is true at an abstract level that what is in the best interests of the profession is also in the best interests of the patient, in practice differences may emerge. I found it useful to think which offences impinged more on the patient or the doctor, the public or the profession. Advertising and canvassing are offences against the profession which are not of real public concern; indeed, restrictions on advertising have now been substantially relaxed by the Monopolies Commission (see Chapter 13), although distinctions are made between GP and specialist advertising. Robbing the health authority, for example by false returns of expenses, is also an offence against the profession, bringing it into disrepute, and against the public in the sense of misappropriating public funds, but of no particular consequence to individual patients so long as the doctor in question treats them appropriately. A drug-addicted doctor is a menace to himself or herself as or well as to her or his patients and may well not be fit to practise; a doctor who prescribes drugs of addiction other than for *bona fide* medical reasons is a menace to his patients and to the public in general; if she or he is not personally addicted the doctor is simply misusing professional power for gain against the interests of others. A doctor who abuses the trust of a patient by seducing or otherwise sexually abusing her or him in the course of treatment or examination is misusing his or her power in the

Table 11.2 Professional discipline 1974

Alleged misconduct or conviction	Cases committees considered			
	Penal cases		Discipline	
	Convictions	?SPM	Convictions	?SPM
Disregard responsibilties to patients	0	5	0	4
Alcohol abuse	38	1	4	0
Drug abuse	5	2	13	1
Non-bona fide prescribing	1	1	3	4
Illegal abortion	0	0	1	0
Improper association/adultery	0	5	0	2
Breach of confidence	0	1	0	1
Dishonesty	13	0	2	5
Violence	5	1	0	0
Indecency	4	0	1	1
Advertising/canvassing	0	3	0	2
False certification	2	1	0	0
False claim to qualification	0	0	0	0
Other charges	7	2	0	0
Total	75	22	24	22

Total complaints/letters received: 847

Some cases involved more than one kind of offence and are shown in more than one column: the table is thus really of charges not cases.
Source: *GMC Annual Report for 1974*, pp. 12–13.

doctor–patient relationship; the action will damage the profession if it becomes known, but the immediate suffering is inflicted on the patient. A doctor who has an affair with a freely consenting patient is in another category, but GMC practices permit enquiry into whether or not this was the case. Failing to visit a patient when reasonably called out, or failing to treat or refer as necessary, may bring the profession into disrepute but are immediate offences against a patient.

For the period 1976–1984 I tried to reclassify charges as shown in Table 11.3, distinguishing between offences principally against the profession and those principally against the public. This may help readers in interpreting tables which follow based on the GMC's classification.

Table 11.3 GMC: A classification of cases of discipline and conduct 1976–1984

1. Drugs:
     by deception etc. for own use
     supplying otherwise than for bona fide treatment
2. Alcohol abuse:
     drunk driving and allied offences
     other drinking offences
3. Forgery, theft and other misappropriation of property:
     from health authority
     from other
4. Offences against patients:
     Sexual;
       improper association
       indecent behaviour
       gross indecency
       indecent assault
     financial;
       improperly charging fees
       other, e.g. extracting loans
     failure to visit, treat, refer,
       mistreatment,
       incompetence
     abuse of confidentiality
     improper delegation
5. Offences against colleagues/the profession:
     advertising canvassing
     improper delegation
     perverting, obstructing justice
     violent behaviour/murder
     illegal abortion
     depreciation of colleagues
     unregistered practice
     improperly obtaining treatment for patient
     evading animal quarantine
     false claims to qualifications
     impersonation

Disposal decisions

How the committees dispose of the cases which come before them is also indicative of the relative importance which is attached to charges. So far as 1974 is concerned, Sir Denis Hill reports that in 66 of the cases the penal cases committee heard, 'warning letters were sent to practitioners following proceedings in the criminal courts or elsewhere in which findings had been made reflecting on the professional conduct of the doctor'. Warning letters were also sent in a further 22 such cases; these will have been sent on the instructions of the president without being referred to the penal cases committee (Hill, 1975, p. 12). In the same year the disciplinary committee heard 46 cases (24 convictions and 22 possible SPMs). Table 11.2 shows the types of cases considered by both penal cases and discipline in 1974.

For the period 1976–1980, the penal cases committee considered 513 cases, as Table 11.4 indicates. Of these 110 were referred to the disciplinary committee; about a fifth of convictions and slightly more of alleged SPM. The greatest number of convictions considered related to the personal abuse of alcohol (38%), followed by convictions for dishonesty (21%) and personal abuse of drugs (15%). Of conviction cases referred, 25% were charges of personal abuse of drugs, 22% of dishonesty, and 17% of personal abuse of drugs. In terms of SPM, 14% of allegations related to disregard of professional responsibility to patients and 15% to misuse of professional power in various ways and 13% for advertising, canvassing and other offences against colleagues. Of these the highest proportion referred to discipline was for the abuse of professional

Table 11.4 Cases considered by penal cases committee and those referred to the disciplinary committee 1976–1980

| | Cases | | | | | |
| | Considered | | | Referred | | |
	Convictions	?SPM	Total	Convictions	?SPM	Total
Disregard prof. responsibility to patients	0	21	21	0	4	4
Misuse of prof. power[a]	0	22	22	0	8	8
Personal abuse						
alcohol	139	1	140	13	1	14
drugs	55	21	76	19	6	25
Non-bona fide prescribing and drugs Act offences	19	17	36	11	6	17
Dishonesty	78	11	89	17	4	21
Violence	9	3	12	0	0	0
Indecency	26	5	31	11	0	11
Advertising/canvassing	0	20	20	0	1	1
False certification						
False qualification	4	8	12	1	1	2
Other	34	20	54	4	3	7
Total .	364	149	513	76	34	110

[a] Abuse, rudeness, improper influence, improper sexual/emotional relationship, breach of professional confidence. In some years some of these may be concealed as 'other' since these headings were not entered every year.
Source: *GMC Annual Reports.*

power (8/22), followed by prescribing other than for bona fide reasons or offences under the 1971 Drugs Act (6/17) and the personal abuse of drugs (6/21).

I sat on the disciplinary committee from 1976 to 1980, when it ceased to exist. During that period the committee dealt with a total of 224 cases. Of these I sat on panels which dealt with 86 cases (42 new; 37 resumed; 7 applications for restoration). Examination suggests that these were reasonably representative of the total. Of the total 224 cases heard, 98 were new cases, about two thirds being convictions and the remainder possible SPM. The committee also dealt with 100 resumed cases and 26 applications for restoration. For that period I have all the data at my disposal and have made a summary of the new cases brought before the committee and the disposal decisions (Table 11.5).

The difficulty the committee had in dealing with the sick doctor is reflected in the heavy use of postponement for drug and alcohol offences in these new cases. At the same time, erasure, frequently forthwith, is most used for this category. For disregard of professional responsibility, such as failure to visit, treat and refer, two out of ten cases were found not guilty. Of those found guilty, one was concluded and one admonished. Suspension was used twice, once forthwith, but erasure not at all.

Table 11.5 New cases and their outcomes: GMC disciplinary committee 1976–1980

					Charge			
Outcome	Drugs	Alcohol	Fraud	Sex	Failure visit/ treat	Against profession	False qualifi- cations	Total
Adjourned	0	1	0	2	1	2	0	6
Not guilty	0	0	0	1	2	1	0	4
Conclude	0	0	0	0	1	0	0	1
Admonish	4	1	9	5	2	1	1	23
Postpone	21	7	3	4	2	1	0	38
Suspend	1	0	4	1	1	0	0	7
Suspend forthwith	3	0	0	1	1	0	0	5
Erase	2	0	1	0	0	1	0	4
Erase forthwith	6	1	0	1	0	1	1	10
Total	37	10	17	15	10	7	2	98

Sources: *GMC Annual Reports*.

Cases and their disposal in the new Council

Figures 11.1–11.3 showed how complaints received moved through the Council in the period 1983–1987. Tables 11.6–11.9 show how the preliminary proceedings and professional conduct committees respectively dealt with the cases sent to them.

Table 11.6 shows that the PPC received 1111 cases in these years, divided almost equally between convictions and alleged SPM. Most cases (259) related to disregard of professional responsibilities, i.e. failure to visit, treat, refer, and all constituted alleged SPM. The second largest category was the personal abuse of alcohol (225), almost all (222) being convictions (these will have had to come to PPC despite the existence of the health committee because all convictions must be considered by the PPC).

Table 11.6 Cases before preliminary proceedings committee 1983–1989

	All cases	Type of case[a]	
		Conviction	Alleged SPM
Disregard of professional responsibility to patients	259	0	259
Dishonesty	131	112	19
Non-bona fide prescribing etc.[b]	82	25	57
Misuse of professional power[c]	65	1	64
Indecency	56	21	35
Canvassing, advertising etc.	69	0	69
Violence	34	28	6
False certification	26	5	21
Improper delegation	5	0	5
False claim to professional experience, qualifications etc.	12	0	12
Attempting to obstruct/pervert justice[d]	10	7	3
Personal abuse			
alcohol	225	222	3
drugs	41	25	16
Other cases (unspecified)[e]	96	53	43
Total	1111	513	598

[a] In reporting cases before the PPC, unlike the PCC, the GMC do not distinguish vases where conviction and SPM may be involved.
[b] Includes offences under the Misuse of Drugs Act.
[c] Includes offences classified by the GMC as improper sexual or emotional relations with patients; using undue or improper influence over a patient; improperly demanding or charging fees; breach of professional confidentiality.
[d] Only listed separately from 1988.
[e] Includes 'other offences' against patients or profession and cases where at professional conduct committee charges fell under more than one head.
Source: *GMC Annual Reports*.

Dishonesty (131) followed, again almost all (112) being convictions. Non-bona fide prescribing of drugs of addiction (not including personal abuse of alcohol which is listed separately) took fourth place (82 cases, 26 involving convictions). Canvassing, advertizing and similar offences against professional colleagues came fifth, all alleged SPM. This is followed very closely by a category I have called misuse of professional power, in which I have included matters such as having improper sexual or emotional relations with a patient, breaches of professional confidentiality, improperly demanding or charging fees and otherwise exercising undue influence over a patient.

Table 11.7 shows the disposal decisions made by the committee classified as follows:

A. No action taken or case adjourned till the following year.
B. Letter of advice or admonition sent; in some but not all years these are distinguished. What was a 'warning letter' in the 1970s has become a 'letter of advice' in the 1980s.
C. Case adjourned *sine die* so that health procedures may be followed (all convictions must come to PPC).
D. Referred to PCC.

The largest number of cases were dealt with by sending a letter of advice or admonition (category B: 44%); a third (33%) were referred to the PCC (category D); in almost a quarter of the cases the committee took no action. This quarter was divided almost equally between category A, where either no action at all was taken or the case was adjourned for a year (12%), and those (category C) which were adjourned *sine die* so that health procedures could be invoked (11%). This last amounts to a positive action: the PPC has determined that, prima facie, the alleged offence, or, in the great majority of cases, conviction (e.g. for drunk driving or drug abuse offences), has occurred because the doctor's health is impaired. So far as category A is concerned, the statistics do not always distinguish between a definitive 'no action' and adjournment. The aggregate can be inferred, however, and overall almost 80% seem to come in the 'no action' category.

The disposal of cases of alleged disregard of professional responsibility to patients is divided almost equally between categories B and D. That is to say, either the cases are referred to the PCC for further enquiry or, when the doctor has admitted the conviction or that there is substance in the charge, she or he is either advised to improve her or his future behaviour or admonished for the offence and reminded that it will be on his or her record to be referred to in case of any future infringements. Some 10% are adjourned or no action is taken; a very few are referred to health. Somewhat in contrast, where the allegation is of misuse of professional power,

Table 11.7 Preliminary proceedings committee 1983–1989[a]

	Type of decision made[b]				
	A[c]	B	C	D	Total
Disregard of professional responsibility to patients[d]	25	113	4	117	259
Dishonesty	6	67	13	45	131
Non-bona fide prescribing etc.[e]	8	17	3	33	61
Misuse of professional power[f]	25	10	1	29	65
Indecency	7	24	3	22	56
Canvassing, advertising etc.	24	27	0	18	69
Violence	6	16	4	7	33
False certification	2	4	0	21	27
Improper delegation	0	1	–	4	5
False claim to professional experience, qualifications etc.	0	6	0	6	12
Attempting to obstruct/pervert justice[g]	0	4	2	3	9
Personal abuse					
alcohol	8[h]	154	54	6	222
drugs	13	15	29	17	74
Other cases	13	35	14	38	100
Total	137	493	127	366	1123

Total (column A) no action 107
Total presumed adjourned   30

[a] In tabulating cases conviction and SPM are not distinguished in GMC reports.
[b] Key: A, No action/adjourned till following year; B, Letter of advice/admonition sent (always distinguished; C, Adjourned *sine die* so that health procedures may be followed; D, Referred to professional conduct committee.
[c] Until 1988 no action or deferred action was reported only in a footnote. Counts are of types of cases, not numbers of practitioners.
[d] Includes four charges in 1989 of irregularities in surgical operation.
[e] Includes offences under the Misuse of Drugs Act.
[f] Includes improper sexual or emotional relations with patients; using undue or improper influence over a patient; improperly demanding or charging fees; breach of professional confidentiality.
[g] Only listed separately from 1988.
[h] One referred to health committee.
Source: *GMC Annual Reports.*

no action or adjournment is a major disposal route: about 38% go this way and about 44% are sent to PCC. This is the only offence category in which no action/adjournment constitutes so proportionately large a disposal route.

False certification, a particular example of the misuse of professional power, stands out as the alleged offence where referral to the PCC is the preferred disposal route (21 out of 27 cases). Over half (33/61) the cases of prescribing other than for bona fide reasons also go to the PCC. Although adjournment *sine die* (referral to the health procedures) is occasionally used for most kinds of alleged offence, it is most often used where the personal abuse of alcohol or drugs is concerned, a relatively few such cases going to PCC.

As Table 11.1 showed, the number of days on which the PCC met increased noticeably from 1983 onwards. In 1986 the number of PCC panels was increased from two to three to accommodate the increased volume of work. This arose less from the increase in practitioners than from a wish to meet public demands for a more vigilant GMC, particularly in areas bordering on competence to practise (see Chapter 13).

So what did the PCC do with the cases that were sent to it? Table 11.8 shows the cases it considered in 1983–1989. The great majority related to disregard of professional responsibility, rather more than a third of all it heard. None of these derived from convictions; all were reported cases

Table 11.8 Cases before the professional conduct committee 1983–1989

	All cases	Types of case		
		Conviction	Conviction and conduct	Alleged SPM
Disregard of professional responsibility to patients[a]	121	0	0	121
Dishonesty	49	42	2	5
Non-bona fide prescribing etc.[b]	46	9	3	34
Misuse of professional power[c]	32	0	2	30
Indecency	18	4	0	14
Canvassing, advertising etc.	15	0	0	15
Violence, including murder	9	5	2	2
False certification	9	5	0	4
Improper delegation	7	0	0	7
False claim to professional experience, qualification etc.	6	0	0	6
Attempting to obstruct/pervert justice[d]	6	2	0	4
Personal abuse				
alcohol	5	3	1	1
drugs	5	2	0	3
Other offences				
against patients[e]	4	1	0	3
against profession[f]	2	0	0	2
Multiple charges[g]	9	0	2	7
Total	343	73	12	258

[a] Includes three charges in 1989 of irregularities in surgical operation.
[b] Includes offences under the Misuse of Drugs Act.
[c] Includes offences classified by the GMC as improper sexual or emotional relations with patients (17); using undue or improper influence over a patient (8); improperly demanding or charging fees (4); breach of professional confidentiality (3).
[d] Includes one case in 1988 of attempting to obstruct the professional conduct committee.
[e] Includes abusive behaviour (2), unauthorized absence from duty (1), false claims to treatment (1).
[f] Includes acquiescing in improper drug use in residence (1); seeking improper inducement to prescribe (1).
[g] Not classified because charges fall under more than one head.
Source: *GMC Annual Reports*.

Table 11.9 Decisions of the professional conduct committee 1983–1989

	Disposal decision								
	A	B	C	D	E	F	G	H	Total
Disregard of professional									
responsibility to patients[a]	46	26	13	12	13	8	3	3	124
Dishonesty	2	13	0	23	9	0	0	2	49
Non-bona fide prescribing etc.[b]	5	11	4	8	15	4	0	0	47
Misuse of professional power[c]	4	6	0	11	7	1	0	1	30
Indecency	5	1	0	4	7	0	0	0	17
Canvassing, advertising etc.	7	7	0	0	0	1	0	0	15
Violence, including murder	0	0	0	1	7	0	0	1	9
False certification	1	4	0	3	1	0	0	0	9
Improper delegation	0	3	0	0	1	0	0	3	7
False claim to professional									
experience, qualifications etc.	0	0	0	1	4	0	1	0	6
Attempting to obstruct/pervert justice[d]	3	0	0	0	3	0	0	0	6
Personal abuse									
alcohol	1	0	0	0	3	0	1	0	5
drugs	1	2	0	1	0	0	1	0	5
Other offences[e]	1	1	0	0	1	0	0	1	4
Multiple charges[f]	1	3	0	1	3	1	0	0	9
Total	77	77	17	65	74	15	6	11	342

[a] Includes three charges in 1989 of irregularities in surgical operation.
[b] Includes offences under the Misuse of Drugs Act.
[c] Includes offences classified by the GMC as improper sexual or emotional relations with patients; using undue or improper influence over a patient; improperly demanding or charging fees; breach of professional confidentiality.
[d] Includes one case in 1988 of attempting to obstruct the professional conduct committee.
[e] Includes abusive behaviour, unauthorized absence from duty, false claims to treatment, acquiescing in improper drug use in residence, seeking improper inducement to prescribe.
[f] Not classified because charges fall under more than one head.
Source: *GMC Annual Reports.*

alleging SPM, as were 30 out of the 32 cases of misuse of professional power, 34 out of 46 cases of non-bona fide prescribing and 14 out 18 cases of alleged indecency. Dishonesty was the largest category where the PCC had to deal with conviction cases. This contrasts with the days before the health procedures were established when convictions related to alcohol and drugs loomed so large.

What the committee did with these cases is shown in Table 11.9. The disposal decisions are categorized as follows:

A. Not guilty of SPM.
B. Admonish or conclude the case.
C. Registration in future to be subject to conditions.
D. Suspension for a defined period.

E. Erasure
F. Adjourned to the following year.
G. Referred to the health committee.
H. Determination postponed.

The new possibility of making registration conditional was used sparingly in this period and then only for disregard of professional responsibility and prescribing for other than bona fide reasons and allied offences.

Of the larger categories of offence it is clear that the PCC experienced the greatest difficulty in finding SPM in cases of disregard of professional responsibilty. Thirty-six per cent of cases heard were found not guilty compared with 13% of other types of offence against patients, 11% in non-bona fide prescribing and offences concerning drugs or 4% in cases of dishonesty. To some extent, but not entirely, this is accounted for by the admission of convictions, which leaves the committee only to decide whether the offence amounts to SPM: the proving of guilt has been done for it. In charges of SPM without conviction the committee has to prove guilt itself.

There is also the question of the disposal decisions reached in cases where the doctor has been found guilty. Looking simply at the proportions of erasures, non-bona fide prescribing and offences against the 1971 Drugs Act attracts the highest proportion of the larger offence categories (20%); disregard of responsibility to patients (failure to visit etc.) follows with 17% and dishonesty with 12%.

However, when one looks at the disposal decisions in terms of the proportions of each meted out to those found guilty (see Table 11.10), it transpires that only 19% of those found guilty of SPM on account of their disregard of professional responsibility to patients were erased during this period, 18% suspended and 38% admonished or the case concluded. This compares with 20% of those charged with dishonesty and found guilty of

Table 11.10 Some disposal decisions in the larger categories of offence (percentages)

	Found not guilty	Of those found guilty:		
		Erased	Suspended	Admonish/conclude
Disregard	36	19	18	38
Non-bona fide prescribing	11	39	21	29
Misuse of professional power	13	28	44	24
Dishonesty	4	20	28	49
All charges	22.5	22	19	22.5

SPM, 49% suspended and 28% admonished or concluded. Readers will recall that suspension was originally brought in to handle cases of 'sick doctors' before the health procedures were introduced. Where SPM was found in drug offences 39% were erased, 21% suspended and 29% admonished. Misuses of professional power, where SPM was found, led to 28% being erased, 44% suspended and 24% admonished.

All in all one is obliged to conclude that although more cases where the patient/public's interest is involved over and against the professional are nowadays considered by PCC, the GMC still finds difficulty in taking them as seriously as offences against the profession and certainly as many members of the public would.

Unfit for health reasons

Since the 1978 Act the routes for the initial disposal of complaints have increased, notably by the addition of the health committee procedures for handling sick doctors. Whereas previously the president had formed the habit of appointing one preliminary screener to aid him in deciding how complaints received should be handled, he now appoints two preliminary screeners, one for conduct (PSC) an one for health (PSH)[1]. Cases are sorted on a prima facie basis as to whether they are conduct or health, the PSC and PSH being able to consult each other and cross-refer.

Sir Denis Hill, who played a large part in the establishment of the health procedures and was appointed the first PSH, explained the procedures at some length in the GMC's *Annual Report* of 1980, the year they were first established, and again in 1981. From 1982, after Sir Denis' death, Dr Connell was appointed PSH. He continued to work in health screening as assistant to Sir John (now Lord) Walton, the president, or as the PSH until 1990. At that time he was able to make a full report to Council of the first ten years of the PSH's work (*GMC Minutes, CXXVII,* 1990, pp. 346–355). Dr Allibone, as chair of the health committee, undertook a similar review of the committee's work over this first decade (*GMC Minutes, CXXVII,* 1990, pp. 360–366).

Of the cases reported to the committee who were invited to be medically examined, over three quarters were alleged to be suffering from drug- and/or alcohol-related problems with in some cases, an admixture of mental illness (485 were reported to Council of whom 311 were invited for examination). The remaining quarter were mentally ill. Only 0.5% of cases involved physical illness alone, although physical illness was also a component in some few of the drug/alcohol/mental illness cases. Of those invited to undergo medical examination, most were between 30 and 60 years old; 15% were women. The doctors were almost equally divided between hospital and general practice (33% and 39% respectively; in contrast to the proportions coming before discipline or conduct); 20% were not working.

The health procedures as established included the health committee, but the GMC's intention was that sick doctors should be dealt with clinically rather than legally; indeed the procedures as finally enacted were necessarily much more formal than Sir Denis had wished. Most cases, therefore, are dealt with by the PSH. As Dr Connell indicates, he considers his main task, having identified possible cases, is to keep them from the committee if possible. When the PSH receives cases for consideration he (always a man up to now) examines the evidence to ascertain whether the doctor reported may be unfit to practice for health reasons. If there is a prima facie case, he invites those doctors to submit to a medical examination. If the doctor agrees, she or he will be examined by doctor drawn from lists of doctors throughout the country. The members of these lists are nominated by the royal colleges and faculties and the BMA through the central committee for consultants and specialists (formerly the central committee for hospital medical services) and the general medical services committee.

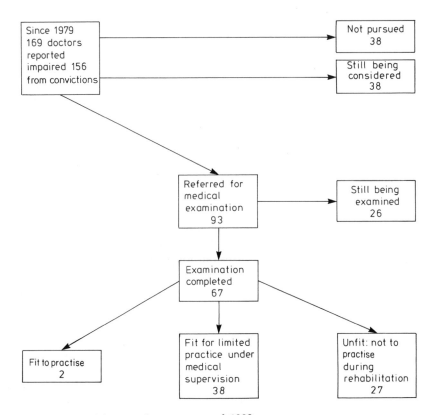

Figure 11.4 Health procedures as at end 1983.
Source: *GMC Annual Report for 1983.*

Most doctors co-operate with the procedures. The great majority of
cases reaching the Council are of doctors whose health is impaired by
reason of alcohol or drug addiction. Examinations take quite some time to
set up and conclude; thus no examinations were complete until the end of
1981. The preliminary screener will only pass cases to the health committee
if either the doctor refuses to co-operate with the procedures and be
examined or, having been examined, she or he is found unfit to practise
and refuses to accept the treatment and/or the restrictions on practice
which have been recommended. I was a member of the health committee
from 1980 to 1984 but it did not meet until 1981 when the first cases
were ready for it. In addition to those passed to it by the preliminary
screener, cases reach the health committee from the PPC and the PCC: see
Figure 11.4.

Ten years of the health procedures

In this review of the ten years, Dr Connell has indicated how the 485 new
cases of alleged unfitness to practise by reason of impaired health have
passed through the system. This is shown in Figure 11.5. In 136 out of the
485 no further action was taken. This may be because the PSH did not consider the evidence amounted to serious impairment or because insufficient
evidence was available and no more was forthcoming The early reports
make plain that sometimes the PSH was prevented from pursuing cases
because the person or authority who initially reported the cases did not
submit adequate evidence or, when asked for further evidence, was unable
or unwilling to provide more. Thus, for example, in 1984 the president
reported that from 1980 onwards the preliminary screener could take no
further action in 47 cases because there was insufficient evidence of serious
impairment or there was inadequate information. This matter was still
worrying the preliminary screener in 1990. He did not take action in 11 out
of 47 cases in 1989–90, in some cases (although it is unclear how many) for
the reason mentioned.

As Figure 11.5 shows, the commonest route was for a doctor to be invited
to attend for a medical examination (311), to agree to submit (266) and to
be examined (262), which was done by a member of the relevant regional
panel. Almost three quarters (165) were judged to have some impairment
but be fit to practise within limitations, such as medical and other supervision. A quarter (65) were found so impaired as to be unfit to practise. Of
those with some impairment the majority (203) accepted the supervision
offered, including the limitations on their practice or the voluntary cessation of practice which was advised. Thus over the years 203 people have
been and 68 are still being medically supervised.

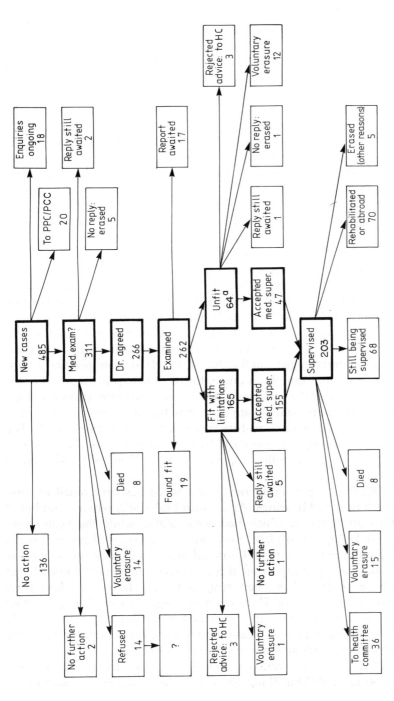

^a There is ambiguity as to whether this is 65 or 64.

Figure 11.5 Doctors' routes through the health procedures: 1980–1990. Source: *GMC Minutes*, CXXVII (1990), pp. 357–359

There are those who have followed a different path. A few (19 in ten years) were found not impaired and fit to practise. Some, at the different stages, have taken voluntary erasure from the register (30 in all). A few have failed to respond and been erased for this and other reasons (11). Seventy are listed as being rehabilitated or having 'gone abroad'; proportions of each are not given. Some (42), because they refused the advice given or were unable to sustain their compliance, were referred to the health committee; others died (16).

None of the examinations or treatment sessions are undertaken by the PSH. They all take place in relevant regions and localities around the country. The PSH runs what he calls a 'paper clinic'. For those who find themselves referred to the health committee, however, the Council premises are the venue, for there the health committee meets.

All the health committee proceedings are *in camera*, so only restricted amounts of information are available about it, but the ten year review is a help. The health committee operates under formal rules with proper representation for the doctor if she or he so wishes, full information being made available to him or her as to the allegations of unfitness which have been made. Initially there was strong resistance to the respondent sick doctors being told their full diagnosis, but this was overcome.

The health committee may suspend a doctor or impose restrictions on practice; it may also postpone a decision or adjourn a hearing on the basis of voluntary undertakings from the doctor, to refrain from practice and/or accept treatment, for example. A doctor found unfit to practise may be suspended for no longer than one year, so those doctors who do not become fit within the year have again to appear before the committee. This, as time has gone by, has come to constitute much of the committee's work. The number of cases being monitored by the committee increased from five at the end of 1981 to 17 the following year, rising to 22 in 1984–1985 and 40 in 1989–1990.

Since 1982 the proportion of new cases heard has been small in comparison with resumed hearings. Apart from 1981–1982, when a number of cases (14) came forward which had accumulated while the health procedure were being put in place, new cases have averaged about seven a year, ranging from four to nine. Resumed hearings include not only those doctors who are appearing to see if their suspensions may be ended, but those whose practice has been restricted, or whose case had been adjourned. In 1989–1990 of 37 resumed hearings, 22 were being resumed for the fourth time (or more—up to eight so far) (see Table 11.11). That table also shows the routes by which cases had reached the committee. Over the decade there were 265 hearings relating to 74 doctors.

Table 11.12 shows the outcomes of all the cases from 1980 to 1990. Perhaps the most striking thing about it is the relatively few number of

Table 11.11 Cases heard by the health committee 1980–1990

Number of meetings		36
Number of hearings		265
New cases considered		
Referred by PSH	54	
Referred by PPC	11	
Transferred from PCC	9	
Total new cases		74
Resumed hearing of cases		
2nd and 3rd hearings	108	
4th or more	83	
Total number resumed		191
Number of cases being monitored in 1990		40

Source: *GMC Minutes, CXXVII,* 1990, pp. 364–365.

Table 11.12 Health committee disposal decisions 1980–1990

Adjourn		
at 1st hearing	17	
subsequently	24	
Total adjourned		41
Serious impairment found		
at 1st hearing	55	
later	147	
Total seriously impaired		202
Conditional registration imposed		
at 1st hearing	17	
later	71	
Total conditional registration		88
Registration suspended		
at 1st hearing	38	
later	82	
Total registration suspended		120
Case concluded by committee		
at 1st hearing	2	
later	18	
Total cases committee concluded		20
Other conclusions[a]	14	
Total other conclusions		14
Total disposal decisions		486

[a] This includes 11 doctors who removed their name from the register at their own request and three who died.
Source: *GMC Minutes, CXXVII,* 1990, p. 364.

cases which the committee has been able to conclude. Of the 52 who were suspended for the first time, 42 were suspended immediately, a measure of how serious 80% of cases were thought to be.

As in conduct the GMC is only concerned with *serious* misconduct so in health it is only concerned with *serious* impairment. A difficulty here is that by the time cases reach the committee the health problem may be resistant to treatment. This accounts for the number of cases in the 'paper clinic' and before the health committee which take a long time to treat or where success is not achieved. There are two problems here. One that practitioners had, and many still have, is difficulty in recognizing that the health procedures were designed to be friendly and supportive to the sick doctor while at the same time protecting the public from those unfit to practise. Consequently there was/is reluctance to report or to follow through with enough information. In many cases the condition is consequently far advanced before the preliminary screener receives it and certainly before it reached the health committee.

The second problem was that other arrangements were needed outside the formal GMC procedures to catch cases of potential serious unfitness at a stage when the condition was more readily treatable. There are some local procedures within the NHS to this end. The GMC felt, however, that more support services were needed, but that it would have been inappropriate for it to try to undertake these along with its statutory tasks. In 1982 the Council consequently began consultative procedures within the profession as to the possibility of setting up a national counselling and welfare service to support doctors who were ill and to help them before things got too serious. A model much before them was a support scheme for anaesthetists set up by the Association of Anaesthetists. By 1984 a steering committee had been set up; by 1987 the GMC's *Annual Report* said that the National Counselling and Welfare Service had become an effective informal alternative to the health committee procedures. Totally separate from the GMC formally and in practice, anyone may ring the service in confidence saying they think they have a problem or they are worried about a colleague.

In concluding his ten-year review Dr Connell referred to this and to his hope that cases will be dealt with earlier. He also indicated that the failure of informants to produce sufficient evidence to enable the health procedures to work properly in all cases continued as a frustration. Furthermore he would like the legislation changed so that the health committee may refer cases back to the informal procedure of the 'paper clinic' where they feel this would be appropriate. Dr Allibone in his conclusion drew attention to the difficulty of finding suitable employment for doctors who had been out of practice for health reasons. They need posts where they could start on limited practice with their work and their health being

carefully supervised. Arrangements are being sought whereby eight super-
numerary posts could be established nationwide for this purpose. Their
establishment depend on central funds being available. Dr Allibone
referred also to the 'daunting social and economic problems' which sick
doctors face in addition to their illness. The health committee are thinking
about a pilot scheme to provide the necessary support as a test of what is
possible.

Discipline in the 1980s and for the 1990s

To conclude—important changes have taken place in the years that I have
reviewed in the way practitioners were disciplined. Notably the differentia-
tion of 'sick' from 'bad' doctors led to more humane procedures from the
doctors' point of view. One hopes in the longer run it will lead to a greater
willingness on the part of the addicted or the mentally ill to seek help and
to better reporting and treatment of the sick. A quite different kind of study
from this would be needed to know whether that is already happening.
There are now a wider range of options available in the disposal of cases.
More cases involving the knowledge, skill and experience, in short the
competence, of the doctor as well as his or her performance were being
brought forward. These, however, were consistently found hard to prove
and even when proved received somewhat lenient treatment compared
with other types of cases. In some ways the procedures themselves are
nowadays better reported and rather more open than they used to be; new
restrictions have, however, been introduced notably on availability of transcripts. The balance of the evidence over these years suggests that offences
against the profession are still taken more seriously than offences against
the public. The sense that this was so led, as the 1980s progressed, to
mounting criticisms of the Council. It his also led the Council itself to
develop proposals for an additional arm, in the shape of performance
reviews, to the disciplinary armoury. These matters will be discussed in
Chapter 13.

   The arrangement which have been discussed in this chapter apply only
to currently registered doctors. These include, as we have seen, a number
of doctors qualified overseas both on limited and full registration. However, those who are *applying for* limited registration are dealt with by a
different procedure which is discussed in the following chapter.

Note

1. More recently a lay screener has also been added.

certain superiors. Arrangements are being sought whereby appropriate monetary costs could be established nationwide for this purpose. Thus establishment demand on central funds being equalized. Doctors referred also to the daunting social and economic problems, which doctors face in addition to their illness. The health community are thinking about a pilot scheme to provide the necessary support as a test of what is possible.

Discipline in the 1980s and for the 1990s

12

Maintaining a Register of the Competent II: Overseas Doctors and Limited Registration

Disciplining overseas doctors

When overseas doctors are registered, whether their registration is full or limited, they are subject to discipline in the same way as UK- or EC-qualified and registered doctors. However, being of good character and conduct is essential before doctors qualified overseas can be registered whether under the former temporary registration arrangements or the present limited registration. Initially, doubts raised about the conduct or character of an overseas doctor were most commonly activated when doctors applied for a further period of the very short term temporary registration. In those circumstances it was effectively through this mechanism that overseas doctors were disciplined. Because these conditions of registration were different from those of UK-qualified doctors, it was decided in 1974 to take all such cases out of the normal disciplinary procedures of the Council and have them dealt with by the overseas committee.

Legal representation is available to these doctors, as it is to UK doctors being heard in the regular procedures, and a legal adviser attends the committee. The overseas subcommittee (now a committee in its own right) considering the cases might be as small as three or four people, although the quorum has now been raised to 5. As has already been pointed out, until 1979 the overseas committee included no overseas-qualified doctor, nor, in the periods reviewed here (1974–1981 and 1982–1985), a woman. In a significant sense, therefore, until 1979 these doctors, unlike UK doctors on discipline charges, were not being tried by their peers; the committee members had all qualified in the UK and all had full registration. 'There but for the grace of God...' only applied in a limited sense.

Cases under this arrangement began to be reported in 1974. Not all cases considered by the overseas committee, nor all doctors to whom the GMC wrote letters of advice or warning, were reported in the *GMC Minutes*. No cases were reported in 1978. References are, however, made in the minutes to cases previously considered by the committee and to cases previously having been warned or otherwise communicated with. Some unreported selection was in operation and some form of preliminary screening. Consequently it is not possible to give a full account of the disciplining of overseas doctors; the process seems even more mysterious than the disciplining of British doctors already discussed. One can therefore only speak about cases reported without knowing what they constituted of the total problem as defined by the GMC.

Between 1974 and 1981, when the new registration arrangements came into place, the subcommittee reported hearing 59 cases relating to 48 doctors, of which four were women (11 hearings related to reconsideration of the same doctors after adjournment, postponement or to hear further reports). Between 1982 and 1985, 40 hearings were reported relating to 31 doctors of whom five were women.

In 1982 there was discussion of the health problems of overseas doctors, not those which might be specific to them as persons qualified abroad but that, as with registered UK doctors, some overseas-qualified doctors applying for further registration ran into disciplinary problems because they were alcohol or drug addicted. From then on such doctors were invited to submit to medical examination by analogy with UK doctors. Cases where health arrangements were invoked were reported as being heard by the subcommittee only when doctors refused to be examined or ceased to co-operate—in a way analogous to appearance before the health committee. No separate health committee or personnel were set up, nor reports made. Technically, at least, in the case of overseas doctors the question was not whether a doctor could be permitted to stay on the register and continue to practise but whether she or he could be permitted to practise at all. However, when a doctor is applying for a further period of registration the importance of this technical distinction fades.

The cases reported come from a wide range of countries, doctors in a few cases apparently qualifying in countries other than their own. Again data relate only to reported cases. The range of countries includes some in the the Middle East, the Indian subcontinent, Africa and South America. European countries were also included before the EC directives came into operation and before countries such as Greece joined.

Of the 59 cases heard between 1974 and 1981, 38 related to convictions, six to false claims to qualifications (including one of personation) while three related to questions of competence. Between 1982 and 1985 convictions constituted only five out of 40 cases. The new limited registration was now in force, restricted to five years in total; charges of unregistered practice predominated—22 out of the 40. Although it was widely known that the clumsy nature of temporary registration led many doctors to practising unregistered for some periods, these cases did not appear in the earlier reports. Between 1974 and 1981 competence to practise was raised in three of the 59 cases; seven of the 40 in the later period related to questions as to the doctor's knowledge, skill and experience to practise. There were two sex charges (one of gross indecency; one indecent behaviour) in the earlier period and two cases of indecent behaviour in the second.

From 1974 to 1981 the most frequent outcome was that the present application for a further period of temporary registration would be granted, subject to satisfactory reports being made available, or that conduct would be reviewed when any further application was made, sometimes including a warning that any further offence would be taken seriously (20/46 first cases). This is in some ways similar to disciplinary admonition for UK-qualified doctors, but contains an element and a threat built into it which, deriving as it did from the very nature of temporary registration, could not be used for those fully registered. Not infrequently in making judgements the chairperson of the committee would stress what a privilege it was to have temporary registration in the UK which the practitioners would do well to respect.

By the end of the period limited registration was being used, which in five cases was permitted to be renewed. In total therefore 25 out of 46 cases were permitted to re-register. In three cases registration was permitted under conditions only. This was an option which did not become available until after 1979 in the disciplining of fully registered practitioners. No action was taken in two cases and three were adjourned. Two were found on examination to be of good character. Eight of the 46 cases were refused further temporary or limited registration (as the case may be).

In the period 1982–1985 limited registration was refused or not renewed in eight out of 31 cases. Eight others were told they could be considered to be of good character but were read a homily as to the inappropriateness of their misdeeds and the need to behave better in future. Registration was restricted in three cases to particular areas of supervised work. Four doctors were forgiven their periods of unregistered practice but had that time taken off the five years limited registration which was legally possible to them. No action was taken in one case and two were adjourned. Three cases were found to be of good character. Medical examination or continued medical supervision was ordered in two cases.

Some trends seem to appear, although numbers are too small and the series too incomplete to provide more than hints. False claims to qualifications or experience seemed always to be dealt with harshly, while in contrast the three cases reported of alleged sexual interference with patients were found not proved. These committees in both periods were composed of men only. Gross indecency with another male, however, led, on the second offence, to the refusal of renewed registration. The phrase 'putting patients at risk' was used only with regard to unregistered practice (these doctors had previously been registered but had failed to renew).

While some of the same principles and prejudices appear in the reports of all these cases as emerge in the cases of the UK qualified, there are a number of features specific to overseas doctors. A greater willingness to recognize that a practitioner is incompetent or otherwise performing badly is demonstrated than in the case of the fully registered. The disciplinary and professional conduct committees do not, of course, have *formal* powers to deal with competence as such, but Chapter 11 showed how reluctant those committees were to define particular examples of incompetence as SPM, which it *is* in their powers to do.

Because overseas practitioners are qualified they are members of the medical club, but because they qualified abroad, come from different cultural backgrounds and are differently pigmented there always seems to be a doubt as to whether they can be full members of the medical 'club'; only a select few ever seem to fully approach that status.

PART 4

THE DECADE OF THE CONSUMER

13

A Patients' Revolt?

The GMC spent time and trouble throughout the 1970s and into the 1980s seeking to improve its disciplinary procedures. The Council came in for mounting criticism nevertheless. Criticism from within the profession suggesting that it did not adequately guard the professional interest was not new. Professional challenges took new turns, however. The Council was not much used to being challenged in the courts and in industrial tribunals, or to being charged with racial discrimination. 'Lay' criticism was not entirely new either—the Council had, after all, had to contend with Bernard Shaw in the 1920s and in the 1970s Rudolf Klein was a vociferous critic of all the professions, making no exception for medicine (Klein and Shinebourne, 1972; Klein, 1973). However, although 'consumers' of health care had become increasingly organized since the Second World War, direct and public criticism from government and from highly articulate members of the public, one in their own ranks, was a new phenomenon.

The radical right, now in political power, was ideologically opposed to the monopoly which the state had effectively granted to the professions, medicine among them. David Green, in his book *Which Doctor?* (Green, 1985), expressed this right radical philosophy so far as medicine was concerned, proposing the replacement of the GMC by lay control. Politically the philosophy was expressed by government in 1988 in its discussion document on restrictive practices (Cm. 331). While this was primarily addressed to commerce and trade and did not mention the professions, it exempted none of them from its strictures. This was followed in the same year by searching enquiries by the Monopolies and Mergers Commission (MMC) into the GMC's restrictive practices: the Office of Fair Trading (OFT) had been enquiring about the GMC guidance on advertising and had finally referred the Council to the MMC. The GMC had originally been set up on the grounds that it would protect patients and potential patients; now it was being challenged in the name of consumer freedom.

Not only right radicals were critical of the GMC, however. In 1982 the way in which the GMC handled the disciplining of a doctor who had allegedly not attended properly to a sick child who subsequently died drew the attention of Nigel Spearing MP, in whose constituency the child had lived. In 1984 he moved a private members bill which sought to add a charge of unacceptable professional conduct to the present single charge of serious professional misconduct. Furthermore, in 1983 Esther Rantzen in a series of TV programmes exposed some bad medical practice and arraigned the GMC for until then permitting such practice to go unchecked. In 1986 the Council appeared before the Select Committee on the Parliamentary Commissioner for Administration which was considering the reports of the Health Service Commissioner (HSC). Finally, in 1988 Jean Robinson, one-time chairperson of the Patients Association and long-time defender of patients' rights, who had been a member of the GMC since 1979, published a diatribe against the Council, *A Patient Voice at the GMC* (Robinson, 1988).

In what follows I shall discuss the content of these various challenges and what impact they may be said to have had/be having on the Council and its workings. A back-drop to the Council's problems was constituted by continual radical reorganizations of the NHS by government—one of which, that of 1989–1990, brought the BMA into serious and bitter dispute with the Secretary of State for Health; additionally there was increasing government pressure towards medical accountability.

The Spearing Bill

Jean Robinson began her critique of the GMC with an account of the case of Alfie Winn (or Turner), the lad in Spearing's constituency who died. He may not have been curable even with the best treatment, but one cannot know, for good treatment he clearly did not get. Alfie's case came first in the series of events I have mentioned. I also shall discuss that case and Nigel Spearing's response to it as my first example of the patient's revolt. When Dr Archer's case came before the PCC (14–15 March 1983) he was charged with failing adequately to examine, treat or arrange hospital treatment for Alfie. The committee found the charges proved but concluded in the chairperson's words as follows:

> Dr Archer: The committee are seriously concerned by the evidence which has been adduced before them in this case. They are disturbed not only by your failure to arrange appropriate specialist treatment for a seriously ill boy who was your patient but also by the poor standard of courtesy which you extended towards the patient's parents. The committee regard such behaviour as below the standard which can be regarded as acceptable in a medical man.
> They have nevertheless felt able to take account of your expression of regret and the representations made on your behalf. The committee have accord-

ingly determined that in all the circumstances you are not guilty of serious professional misconduct in relation to the facts proved against you in the charge. That concludes the case.

GMC Minutes, CXX (1983), pp. 95–96

This pronouncement may have concluded that case in a judicial sense, but the decision started a train of events not yet concluded. The outcome was of a piece with those which, when I served on the disciplinary committee, I found 'surprising', as I noted in the last chapter. The Archer verdict was one of a number which, when I analysed the records for the first half of the 1980s and noted that more cases of failure to treat, visit or refer were coming from PPC to PCC, also caused me surprise. They suggested that although the GMC were now prepared to look at more cases bordering on the clinical, errors in practice did not rank as seriously in the committee's mind as some other offences (advertising, for example). In the pronouncement on Dr Archer's case I note that the doctor' rudeness was ranked along with his clinical incompetence. That the case did not pass into the records unnoticed by almost all except the aggrieved parents had to do with the following circumstances: Alfie had a determined and strong mother; Nigel Spearing was advising her; Alfie was well known in E16 because he was the mascot of West Ham United Football Club. Furthermore, Dr Archer appeared before the PCC the following year on another serious charge. This time he was found guilty of SPM and referred to the health committee (*GMC Minutes, CXXI*, 1984, pp. 113–114). Dr Archer's illness had not been spotted, or if spotted not reported, sooner than this by anyone.

Nigel Spearing began correspondence with the GMC in 1983 even before Alfie's case had reached the PCC. He formed the opinion that if Dr Archer's behaviour in that case could not be defined as SPM then there should be a lesser charge of unacceptable medical conduct—a phrase used in the PCC's judgement. The New Zealand and a number of other Councils already used these two levels of charge, so there were models. Not being satisfied with the GMC's response in a series of letters and discussions, in 1984 Nigel Spearing moved an amendment to the 1983 Medical Act to introduce this second level of charge. He felt it would increase the power of the GMC to control doctors, giving them an opportunity, for example, to impose condition on a doctor's registration where his or her practice might endanger the public but the known offences could not be judged as SPM.

The GMC response was to set up a working party to consider: (i) the standards against which the conduct of doctors is judged in relation to neglect or disregard of professional responsibilities to patients and in relation to other matters; (ii) the use by the PCC of its power to impose conditional registration. In the meantime it issued press releases and notes for MPs in defence of its position. The working party had discussions with Nigel Spearing but were not convinced by his arguments, which included the point that in its sifting procedures the Council was already making decisions about the seriousness of admitted offences, albeit not in public. When it reported in November 1984, the working party reaffirmed the Council's opposition to two standards of charge. Their arguments were: (i) that two levels of offence might lead to the lesser charge resulting in a more severe penalty than the greater charge; (ii) that there would be judicial difficulty in maintaining a fair and consistent standard between the two charges; (iii) that it would lead to a lowering of standards because defence lawyers would always try to reduce an SPM charge to the unacceptable conduct charge; (iv) there were adequate powers already.

This last argument, that the bill was unnecessary because the GMC already had an adequate range of powers, had some strength. The point, however, is that the Council had never been willing to exploit these powers to the full in cases of patient care bordering on clinical autonomy. In their review of the work of the PCC, the working party confirmed my judgement, recorded in the last chapter, that 'difficulty has most frequently arisen in determining whether the alleged facts justified reference for public inquiry or whether the proven facts amounted to serious professional misconduct' in some of the cases where the allegation is that 'a doctor has disregarded or neglected his professional responsibilities to patients' (*GMC Minutes, CXXI*, 1984, p. 310). A virtue of the Spearing amendment would be to force the Council to consider more such cases, rather than only referring those where it looked as if a charge of SPM could be sustained. Furthermore, the GMC would have to consider these kinds of cases more seriously.

This the working party accepted, but it recommended a different route. It proposed that the 'blue book' of guidance to practitioners should include clearer and stronger advice about the standards of acceptable practice with particular reference to the treatment of patients (*GMC Minutes, CXXI*, 1984, pp. 310–311). The strength of the Council's objections to the 'two standards' does not seem to be matched by the strength of their arguments against the Spearing proposal. Professor David Cole, Dean of Medicine in the University of Auckland and deputy chairperson of the New Zealand Medical Council, could not comprehend the strength of the GMC's objections. He was used to working with different levels of misconduct and thought the GMC was missing an opportunity. Jean Robinson's suggestion that the Council could not bear the thought of being legislated for on the basis of a lay private member's bill does seem plausible. Neither the Houses of Parliament nor the civil service formerly concerned themselves very much with the workings of the GMC (or any of the other professions), but times had changed.

Challenge from the Privy Council

In the meantime a dispute had arisen between the GMC on the one hand, and the Privy Council (PC) and the departments of health on the other. In 1984 the GMC had sought to improve the procedure rules of the fitness to practise committees (PPC, PCC and health) for experience had shown that the rules made after the reform of the GMC could do with some refinement. New procedures were drafted and submitted, as was routine, to the PC for their approval as well as to medical practitioners (*GMC Minutes*, *CXXI*, 1984, pp. 182–207). The PC for this purpose is effectively composed of the relevant ministers. However, the PC and the departments of health were not inclined to accept the changes proposed, but wanted to see more radical change, including statutory changes along the lines of the Spearing Bill. At this juncture, therefore, the wires became crossed between the Spearing initiative and what had been an apparently routine manoeuvre by the GMC.

It was clear that the public anxieties which lay behind the Spearing Bill could not be brushed off. The president, Sir John (now Lord) Walton, saw the Lord President of the Privy Council and the Chief Medical Officer (CMO) of the Department of Health early in 1985. The working party which had been set up in 1983 to make the original proposals for rule change was reconstituted in February 1985 to consider the results of the consultations. Meantime the president proceeded to consult privately and widely with the royal colleges and other medical organizations about ways in which the Council might meet the criticisms which lay behind the Spearing Bill. He was clearly convinced that the Council could no longer sidestep the issue of discipline and competence to practise. To maintain a register of the competent was the prime task of the Council: serious allegations had been laid that it was not doing this task properly. Government shared those views. The CMO will have conveyed to the president how seriously the matter was being taken by Ministers (*GMC Annual Reports for 1984*, pp. 182–207; *1985*, pp. 270–272; *1986*, pp. 236–271, 429–432; *1987*, pp. 305–308; *1988*, pp. 255–290).

By 1988 agreement had been reached on a number of aspects of the procedure rules, but the major issue of how to handle incompetence remained outstanding—the working party had not yet completed its work. From the outset John Walton had been thinking in terms of some arrangement similar to that of the health committee and its associated local procedures. In the 1989 annual report the new president, Sir Robert Kilpatrick, was able to announce that the new proposals would shortly be unveiled. The basic Walton model has been worked on all the years since. Competence has, however, become performance along the way—but more of that anon. A long road had been travelled since Alfie's unfortunate death in 1983, but Nigel Spearing's bill is not yet dead (1991). He continues his attempts to get it before the House and beyond its first reading.

Esther Rantzen and medical competence

In 1983 Esther Rantzen, on her BBC TV programme *That's Life*, exposed the private practice of a Dr Frempong, a UK-qualified doctor, who was operating on patients using laser surgery to remove tattoos. Patients were left with damage from these operations which led some of them to go to other doctors to have the problems resolved. In the course of five transmissions Esther Rantzen pursued the GMC for failing to check this doctor's practice.

She and the investigatory journalists who were working with her met with the president and Dr Macara to discuss her allegations against the GMC. The way Esther Rantzen went about the problem, exposing it on TV, and her apparent aggression against the GMC, roused members' anger. Nevertheless the Council, following the advice of its executive committee, effectively accepted two major criticisms made on the programme. The first is that, although the GMC 'is not ordinarily concerned with errors in diagnosis or treatment', a practitioner could be said to have 'wilfully disregarded his professional responsibilities to an extent justifying the institution of preliminary proceedings against him' if he persists 'in a branch of practice in which he is clearly incompetent' (*GMC Minutes*, CXX, 1983, App. VIII, pp. 245–246). The guidance in the blue book was modified to take this into account.

The second criticism was that other practitioners were aware of the damage Dr Frempong had done—they had seen and could testify to the results—but had not reported Dr Frempong to the GMC. The doctors were apparently afraid to do so in case they should thereby fall foul of the ethical guidance of the Council about not defaming or depreciating colleagues. Because the practice in question was private, no other disciplinary body could be involved unless patients sued for damages through the courts. The Council resolved to inform registered practitioners in the next *Annual Report* that 'there may be circumstances in which it would be the responsibility of doctors to report to Council evidence which may be regarded as raising a question of serious professional misconduct by a professional colleague'.

Dr Frempong's case came before the PCC in March 1984 (*GMC Minutes*, CXXI, 1984, pp. 91–92). He was charged with SPM on the grounds that in the course of treating two private patients he had caused a skin condition requiring extensive reparative treatment, and that he had advised one of the patients in question not to report to a hospital about the problem; further, he had persisted in a branch of medicine in which he had demonstrated he did not have appropriate knowledge, skill and experience; finally, he had disregarded his professional responsibilities for his patients. Ironically, the question about persisting in a branch of medicine in which he lacked competence (an unethical practice now enshrined in the blue book) was found not proved; all the other charges were proved and Dr Frempong's name was directed to be erased from the register. He appealed to the Privy Council without success. His application to be restored to the register in July 1986 failed, but he was restored in November 1988.

The Sharp and Sultan affair

The 'laser case' was shocking to the public who saw the exposé on TV, but even more upsetting revelations came later. I shall mention two. In 1989, an investigative journalist, Duncan Campbell, again with a TV programme behind him, exposed the case of two doctors, Sharp and Sultan. From 1986 or 1987 they had been conning AIDS patients that they had a remarkable cure and attracting these sufferers as private patients. Sharp and Sultan had no such cure, but 'more than 30 patients with AIDS, cancer, or leukaemia were charged thousands of pounds and given the treatment at the [private] London Bridge Hospital' (Smith, 1989a).

Duncan Campbell (Campbell, 1989) demonstrates that many doctors knew, but did nothing about, this piece of charlatanism. Finally, early in 1989 'a patient and a junior doctor who had watched this extraordinary quackery with mounting anxiety helped instigate the press investigation of Sharp's scientific credentials and medical methods' (Campbell, 1989). They did not go to the GMC, and neither had others before them. This was partly, argues Campbell—and Richard Smith's *BMJ* editorial does not disagree—because the GMC in its blue book then said that 'it is improper for a doctor to disparage, whether directly or by implication, the professional skill, knowledge or qualification or services of any other doctor ... such disparagement may raise a question of serious professional misconduct' (section 65). According to Campbell two doctors whom he and his colleague consulted took legal advice or advice from the GMC 'and were quickly counselled to say nothing at all' (p. 1172). Another clinician 'withdrew completely the public comments he had been willing to make after the GMC and his medical defence society had explained section 65' (p. 1172). However, as Richard Smith points out, the blue book also says that 'a doctor has a duty, where circumstances so warrant, to inform an appropriate body about a professional colleague whose behaviour may have raised a question of serious professional misconduct'.

The advice given to doctors over the Sharp and Sultan case is not the only evidence that the GMC gives more weight to collegial solidarity than to the second duty of reporting those who may be a danger to the public. In 1990 Jean Robinson proposed that the Council should delete section 65 so that doctors were not thereby inhibited from reporting colleagues who they felt were unfit to practise, as indeed a following section indicates they should. The Council did not feel able, or at least not yet, to remove or amend section 65. This may imply that as well as the common reluctance to shop colleagues, whether for conduct or health reasons, there is a strong wish to keep the club together and to impose a duty so to do. Raanan Gillon opened a debate in the *Journal of Medical Ethics* on this topic in September 1990 (Gillon, 1990). The debate was not taken up in the pages of that journal, but the GMC amended its guidelines (GMC (1991), p. 16, paragraphs 62–64) in November 1990 so that paragraph 65 has been replaced (see Chapter 16, 'Conflicts between "brotherhood" and service' for a more detailed discussion).

Kidneys for sale

A further dramatic case of malpractice was yet to be exposed before the 1980s were out; particularly unsavoury—and, sadly, thus newsworthy—it was the subject of an inquiry by the Bloomsbury Health Authority early in 1989. The case had been brought to light by Amin Saliba, the Lebanese-born owner of the Medical Centre International London Clinic, rather than by any medical colleagues, and was exposed by a Sunday newspaper. It reached the GMC disciplinary committee at the end of the year, where it created a record in terms of the length of the hearing: 35 days to complete, days which were spread from early December 1989 until April 1990. A Harley Street physician, a Guy's Hospital urologist and a Dulwich Hospital transplant surgeon had treated fee-paying patients in the private Wellington Humana Hospital in London. They were charged with serious professional misconduct in so far as they were involved in the buying and selling of kidneys for transplant and in certain irregularities which also involved NHS patients and services.

An Act to ban all commercial dealings in human organs was passed in 1989 as a result of the revelations, but the doctors had not been convicted in the courts; they were on SPM charges. Their offences antedated the Act. From 1985 the GMC had warned that

it is unethical and improper for a registered medical practitioner, wittingly or unwittingly, to encourage or to take part in any way in the development of

... trafficking in the sale of human organs ... no surgeon should undertake the transplantation of a non-regenerative organ from a living donor without first making due enquiry to establish beyond reasonable doubt that the donor's consent has not been given as a result of any form of undue influence.'

GMC Minutes, CXXII (1985), App. XVII, p. 338

Nevertheless, with the help of accomplices, advertisements had been placed for kidney donors in Turkey in 1987 and Turkish citizens brought to England to sell their kidneys here. Four of them had been paid between £2500 and £3360 for their kidneys (although the advertisement was said to have offered £10,000 for a kidney). It was alleged, among other things, that the kidney sellers were not told the truth about what would happen to them or in whom their kidneys would be implanted, and further that they were not well cared for during and after their operations. The case received blow by blow press coverage.

At the end of this long trial all three doctors were found guilty of SPM. Raymond Crockett, the Harley Street physician, who had apparently orchestrated the whole affair and benefited particularly from it, was struck off the register; Michael Bewick, the surgeon, and Michael Joyce, the urologist, were allowed to continue to practise subject to conditions.

This case of unethically practising medicine for personal gain, or one might say treating medicine as a commercial activity, happened in the heyday of Mrs Thatcher's enterprise society when government was encouraging the expansion of private medicine and for-profit hospitals were being developed—new for the UK, where private medicine had traditionally been run on a provident basis. Other examples, less dramatic, of the money-making ethos, came before the GMC, such as, for example, that of Dr Mary, who promised to prescribe particular drugs if he was regularly given good lunches by their manufacturers (*BMJ* (1988), 297:313–314). He was brought to book not by other doctors or by patients, but by the pharmaceutical industry itself, no doubt anxious, in view of increasing consumer sensitivity about prescription drugs, to keep its nose clean.

Right radicalism claims to champion the consumer

There was, however, a well-developed ideology behind the 'enterprise society'; so far as medicine was concerned, it found expression in the little-noticed book by David Green *Which Doctor?* (Green, 1985) from the right radical think-tank. This not only proposed the abolition of the GMC and its replacement by a lay controlling body, but also argued for market control of health care.

Like many others on the left as well as the right, Green was convinced that professionals had too much power. In his view this was a result of 'unwise government intervention', not only in granting monopoly privileges (as the 1858 Medical Act did), but also in the very creation of the NHS itself. Restoring the market would allow the consumer to shop around and also permit the extension of alternatives to biomedicine. However, even Green did not propose total deregulation: he was sufficiently impressed with the difficulties of applying the 'buyer beware' principle to health matters, a service in which maltreatment may result in death or irreparable damage—such 'damaged goods' cannot be returned for replacement. Regulation, however, should be minimal.

The body which would replace the GMC should be principally responsible for reviewing training requirements (including whether the knowledge purveyed by training programmes is justified) and maintaining a register of approved courses. This would be a main aid to preventing incompetence. Green was convinced that the GMC's register is not a register of the competent. The new body would also decide which drugs could be available on prescription only. Any rulings made would be registered as restrictive practices and regularly reviewed. The body should have no role in enforcing a code of conduct.

Legal immunities presently enjoyed by medical practitioners should be withdrawn, and nor should there be a state medical service in which jobs are reserved for practitioners licensed by the state. Green called for a 'radical and direct assault on restrictive practices', including entry restrictions, restriction of competition, and, of course, the NHS itself. Of these he especially disliked entry restrictions; qualifications should be reviewed by non-medical people as a guide to consumers.

Although the government have not gone so far as David Green proposed, his work expressed the market ideology behind the enquiries by the Office of Fair Trading (OFT), the subsequent referral of the GMC to the MMC, and the introduction of simulated markets into the NHS, presaged in the 1989 NHS Review (Cm. 555): a package of actions which many doctors have been resisting ever since.

The OFT enquiries

Government, however, did not propose a direct assault on the GMC: it was much more engaged with the NHS. Rather government used existing bodies to challenge some of the GMC's hallowed practices in the name of the free market and of consumer choice. The desirability of further relaxing advertising restrictions was mentioned in the white paper *Promoting Better Health* (HMSO, 1987). In that year OFT began to ask the GMC about restriction on advertising on two grounds: to increase competition among doctors (the ideological one) and to provide patients and potential patients with more information about medical services and practices (something which some patients' organizations had been arguing for for a quarter of a century). On top of this came the restrictive trade practices consultative document—again with the aim of increasing competition—which (shocking to say) included professions like medicine along with all the other trades.

The GMC had just, in 1986, finished a major review of its professional guidance, including that on advertising, and had published a new blue book in 1987. Council was not at all keen to change it again so soon and said so: it felt it had already gone out of its way to meet consumer demands. The new guidance did increase patient protection proportionately to professional protection (Stacey, 1990), but it had not loosened up advertising as much as ministers wanted. Council also drew particular attention to the vulnerability of the sick to persuasive influence, their possible irrationality and their consequent need for protection. The pressures from OFT were to be 'protested vigorously' (*GMC Minutes*, CXXV, 1988, pp. 215–216).

The protests were in vain: in May 1988 OFT reported the GMC to the MMC for investigation under the Fair Trading Act 1973 so far as its agreements and practices relating to advertising were concerned. Council now also found itself dealing with the Department of Trade and Industry (DTI) with regard to the consultative document on restrictive practices, rather than the familiar Department of Health. I understand this has not, however, been taken further. Some recognition continued to be given to the professional status of medicine, as in the phrase the GMC was to quote more than once from the 1987 white paper which said advertising 'should be subject to proper safeguards for the professional status of the practitioners and for the protection of the public'. In reality, however, and notwithstanding their successful nineteenth century escape into professionalism, medicine way now, in government eye at least, a trade.

The GMC and the MMC

In responding to the MMC, the GMC (*GMC Minutes*, CXXV, 1988, App. XII) drew a clear distinction between 'the provision of information about doctors for the benefit of patients and others' and 'promotional activities designed to gain the largest possible market share for an individual doctor or group' (p. 307). The former it had agreed to and even encouraged in its 1987 version of the blue book; the latter 'carries significant dangers', the Council claimed, 'both for individual patients and for the community as a whole' (pp. 307–308).

It was, the Council argued, the inappropriateness of the 'buyer beware' principle for medical services and not the protection of the profession that led it to recommend restrictions on advertising. The restrictions that remained were necessary to preserve the NHS itself and the referral system. The referral system implies that, since the public have direct access to GPs and have to choose for themselves which GP to attend, they should be given information about GPs. This the new GMC guidelines provided for. The public in general do not have direct access to specialists; they are referred by GPs, and it is therefore the GPs and not the public who should have information about specialist services. Here the specialist register would also be important.

The Council felt it important to preserve the referral system in the public interest and gave illustrations of symptoms which might lead patients to the wrong type of specialist—thus wasting time and money, his or her own, the state's or the insurance company's. Evidence was drawn from the USA where attempts were being made to restrict direct public access to specialists. (In passing, one might note that historically in Britain the institutionalization in 1948 of the referral system as part of the NHS had finally settled a century-old dispute between hospital consultants and GPs about access to patients.)

So far as the NHS was concerned, the Council felt that the NHS and market forces—and thus unrestricted competition also—were incompatible with each other. Not then aware of how far the government would go to bring market forces into the NHS, the GMC correctly argued (*GMC Minutes, CXXV*, 1988, p. 310) that the (then) structure of the NHS of itself diminished the application of market forces (exactly why Green disliked it so much). The importance of sustaining the NHS as it then was is taken as self-evident rather than argued in the Council's response to the MMC.

While their enquiries had shown a demand for more information, the Council reported, they had detected no demand for increased competition as such. In these enquiries undertaken for the 1985 review of the GMC guidance on advertising the Council had taken account of patients' as well as professional opinions as expressed through various organizations. (So far as patients were concerned this was a change from what would have happened 15 or even five years earlier.) Patients' organizations had insisted on the need for more information about practitioners and the Council had agreed. However, neither patient nor consumer organizations had argued, the response stated, that doctors should be able to advertise in newspapers or otherwise promotionally in order to increase competition.

Council invoked the ignorance and vulnerability of sick, and particularly of seriously or mentally ill, patients in support of the need for restrictions on promotional or persuasive advertising. The response exhibits distrust of patients' satisfaction with treatment as a reliable indicator of the quality of service (*GMC Minutes, CXXV*, 1988, p. 318). Promotional advertizing would furthermore destroy, Council argued (p. 320), the trust between doctor and patient; even without direct disparagement of others, it would imply that some doctors were not fully competent, thereby reducing the trust of patients in doctors generally. The existence of public trust in the competence of doctors in general was assumed.

In conclusion the GMC's response to the MMC argued strongly for impartial information being made available about practitioners and their services by independent authorities or organizations. It argued equally strongly against any increase in competition and its associated promotional or persuasive advertising.

The MMC (Cm. 582) were not, however, convinced that there were adequate grounds for restricting advertising as much as the GMC wished— there was an element of unjustified monopoly which was against the public interest. Some aspects of the GMC's submission were, however, accepted: advertising should not be of a character which could bring the profession into disrepute; it should not abuse the trust of patients or exploit their lack of knowledge; it should be factual, legal, decent, honest and truthful and should not disparage other doctors or make claims of superiority for the service of the doctor advertised; no explicit or implicit claims to cure particular diseases should be made; canvassing and associated practices should remain banned. Specialists were not to advertise to the public but specialist associations should be able to offer information, if asked, about their members and their qualifications (this had particular significance for worries, for example, about cosmetic surgery, slimming and baldness clinics).

The GMC were given six months to amend their guidance on advertising. The BMA had to amend its ethical guidelines. In a *BMJ* leader (Havard, 1989b), Dr John Havard, who has long experience of medical ethics both at the BMA and the GMC, argued that the MMC had failed to understand the nature of the doctor–patient relationship within which self-promotional advertising is inconsistent with the philosophy of a caring profession. He suggested further that the exemptions which the MMC had found it necessary to introduce because of the limitations of 'buyer beware' in medicine would be difficult to police. Nevertheless the profession had expected some such outcome 'in today's political climate'.

In May 1990 the GMC 'approved revised guidance on the advertising of doctors' services in the UK, significantly relaxing its policy on the matter' as Donald Irvine put it (Irvine, 1991). He wrote as chair of the GMC committee on standards of professional conduct and on medical ethics, rehearsing the whole history of the debates and the changes since 1985. Acknowledging that some doctors do not like these changes any more than they had liked the relaxations of 1987 he concludes:

> I believe that the Council's policy as it now stands represents a reasonable development of those earlier changes, and that it shows the regulatory body

of the medical profession in the UK able to respond both to changes in the way medicine is practised and to criticism of established attitudes which no longer stand up to detailed scrutiny.

Not a trade?

The GMC response to the MMC was made in September 1988. In October Council's comments on the consultative document on restrictive practices were submitted to the DTI (*GMC Minutes, CXXV*, 1988, pp. 331–338). The Council expressed themselves as 'disappointed that the consultative document appears not to distinguish between the carrying on of trades and businesses and the practice of a profession', particularly medicine which Council claimed was not only different from trade but from all other professions. This was why there were restrictions—to protect the public, not the profession. Council also regretted the failure of the consultative document to take full account of the public interest, especially of public health and safety.

The arguments about the control of advertising as being necessary in the public interest, were rehearsed again. Special attention was paid to the referral system and its ethical, practical and financial importance. Having drawn attention to the particular difficulties that would be created if the referral system were prohibited or undermined in any prospective legislation, Council warned that in the public interest, it would be likely to seek a block exemption for registered medical practitioners. A back-drop to these anxieties was, of course, the proposal for the legal profession to reduce the distinctions between solicitors and barristers.

A patient voice at the GMC

1988 was undoubtedly a rough year for the GMC. Not only did it have to deal with OFT, MMC and the DTI, but it also had court cases on its hands: a hitherto unheard of challenge in the courts by Dr Sidney Gee to prevent the PCC from hearing allegations against him; a challenge by Dr Goba before an industrial employment tribunal under the Race Relations Act (in which he was backed by the Commission for Racial Equality); and a case in the High Court in which a Dr Colman unsuccessfully claimed the GMC's guidelines on newspaper advertisements were unreasonable. In this chapter, however, I am not concerned with professional challenges to the GMC's legitimacy but with the increasing outspokenness of patients and their representatives and of government in the 'consumer' interest.

In 1988 Health Rights published the insider's critique of the GMC written by Jean Robinson (Robinson, 1988). The book was published without prior warning to members or officers, thus breaking most of the unwritten rules of the 'club'. Essentially a democrat, Jean Robinson was totally unimpressed by the merits of these unwritten rules whereby gentlemen traditionally run their affairs (c.f. Paxman, 1991).

Jean Robinson had been active in the health arena for many years. One time chairperson of the Patients' Association, she had had long experience of working with patients who were alleging experience of wrongs at the hands of the medical profession. She is perhaps most often thought of in this capacity. She came to the GMC as a nominee of the Association of Community Health Councils for England and Wales. However, her reputation does not only derive from her work as a patients' advocate. She is a careful and highly respected researcher in occupational health, in, for example, asbestos-related disease and cervical cancer; she regularly lectures to medical students and practitioners as well as to those interested in environmental medicine. She has a detailed understanding of the ethics of medical research. She is an energetic campaigner for improved health and health care on a broad front, including for medical practitioners themselves.

Jean Robinson's critique of the GMC is wide-ranging, covering many issues including, for example, those relating to education and overseas doctors. However, Health Rights, she reports, had commissioned her to write particularly about the GMC complaints procedures, so it was to the disciplinary activities of the Council and issues to do with ensuring competence to practise in that she paid most attention. Her extensive experience of all aspects of the consumer complaints procedures—the family practitioner committees (as they then were), the hospital complaints procedure, the health ombudsman and the courts, so far as patient claims for damages are concerned—had shown her at first hand the complex issues and processes involved. She was also familiar with the consequences for patients and their relatives of medical accidents and medical incompetence, not only of the trauma itself but consequences deriving from the way the complaints were handled.

Her main attack on the Council, for such it was, was upon its disciplinary procedures. In a sense she was looking on the Council as a crucial, and the oldest, part of the health treatment complaints mechanism and the only one short of the courts so far as private patients are concerned. This is not how the profession viewed the GMC: most saw its education function as primary. Jean Robinson, very reasonably, took at face value the statutory responsibility of the Council to maintain a register of the competent (as had Merrison) and argued that it did not do that. In particular she castigated Council for hiding, as she saw it, behind the NHS procedures. The standing instructions whereby complaints about NHS treatment are referred back to the complainant with the suggestion that they direct them to the relevant NHS authority had saved the Council much time and money. It had also meant, she argued, that many complaints had not been properly looked at.

In any case, she continued, the NHS procedures had so many weaknesses that they were not a competent way of handling complaints; they constituted a very shaky basis for the GMC to rely on. Furthermore, their weaknesses increased the importance of the GMC's work. This was particularly true of the hospital complaints procedures, whose weakness, she argued, explained why relatively few hospital doctors compared with GPs appeared before the PCC. The GP system was better because GPs were in contract with the state, but it was also limited by that.

She made many criticisms of the GMC's preliminary screening process, particularly that the President could be preliminary screener; he 'should be above, and outside, the disciplinary procedure' she said (Robinson, 1988, p. 14). The job would be better done by a small committee which would include lay members. She was sympathetic to the proposal in the Spearing Bill of more than one level of charge, because that would mean that the GMC would be forced to look at more cases, cases which might be a danger to the public. She does not accept that the letters of advice which the PPC can send when a doctor has admitted an offence constitute an appropriate second level of discipline. She was also particularly concerned that complainants were not informed when warning letters were sent to a doctor in consequence of a complaint. Referring to one case she knew where the GMC had, she alleges, refused to tell the complainant what the outcome of his complaints was; she said 'As a Council member I felt ashamed.' She expressed surprise that the GMC did not have its own investigation unit and is unhappy about the extent to which Council effectively relies on the Departments of Health and the Home Office to pass cases on.

Initially, Jean Robinson served on the PPC, but then she was appointed to the PCC, thus seeing two aspects of the disciplinary work of the Council. She acknowledges that all members of the committee try to do an honest job within the rules but feels they, in the end, 'merely become instruments for the occasional ritual sacrifice' (Robinson, 1988, p. 19).

Her diligence and her connections with community health councils led her to detailed involvement with some difficult cases. She reported one or two where she felt that matters had not been right. In the course of her enquiries she found that the transcripts of hearings which had formerly been readily available to members were now no longer available (Robinson, 1988, pp. 24–26). (See also my experiences noted in Chapter 1.) Only those who had been a party to the hearings could see the transcripts; furthermore, it later transpired that the GMC had decided not to have the proceedings of hearings where the doctor had been found not guilty transcribed at all. Any party to such a hearing wishing a transcript would have to pay for the transcription—a costly matter. Jean Robinson was concerned not only at this change but also that it had been made without discussion in committee or Council—an undemocratic and therefore incorrect procedure to her mind. The new ruling was explained to me as being because the Council did not want hearings which had been concluded to be 'rerun' outside the Council chamber. Jean Robinson reports receiving little support from fellow members when she tried in open Council to improve access to transcripts.

Jean Robinson also reported concern that in the majority of cases considered by the PPC or PCC the initial complainant was unaware of what wag going on and was not called upon as a witness. This was because the 'complainant' was the government's health department to which cases had come via the (then) FPC or through hospital complaints; that was when the department reported that, for example, a GP had been 'fined' for some breach of contract which a patient or patient's relative had originally brought to light. She advised such people to send a report of the local proceedings directly to the GMC themselves so that they might become the 'complainant' and be involved in the Council proceedings. (In subsequent practice they have not necessarily been so treated.) She pointed out that the question of SPM is a different one from breach of contract and may require different, or different presentation of, evidence.

Some of those things which Jean Robinson advocated have now come about. She complained that she failed to get patients' organizations included on the list of bodies to be consulted by the GMC. However, as mentioned above, such organizations have been included in recent rounds of consultation. Lay members are on more committees now, and more of them are included on conduct. One of her major concerns was that 'the GMC seems to have no power over the doctor who does a consistently lousy job'. Furthermore, in her view, it 'is the way doctors behave after a mistake has been made which causes most criticism and really brings the profession into disrepute' (Robinson, 1988, p. 33). The GMC is now about to unveil its 'performance reviews'; whether they will satisfy patients' organizations and persons such as Jean Robinson remains to be seen.

In her conclusion Jean Robinson asked 'will the GMC change?'—a good question. She did not herself suggest a model for change. Throughout her book she referred to reforms in procedure and practice which she felt necessary, many of which she had proposed but, at the time of writing, had failed to achieve. Unlike David Green (and the Medical Practitioners' Union of the mid-1970s) she did not suggest wholesale abolition. She observed that

it is the fact that a new player has entered the game which has caused such a frisson in Hallam Street. The House of Commons, represented by the Labours—Conservative duo of Nigel Spearing and Sir Anthony Grant, is the

real challenge. Powers that Parliament gave are powers that Parliament can
take away. (Robinson (1988), p. 41)

Her parting shot referred to the radicalization which patients have
undergone since the NHS was first established. She is convinced that this
radicalization is not the result of bad care, but has been brought about 'by
the defensive and sometimes dishonest reactions of doctors and health
authorities when complaints were made' (Robinson, 1988, p. 41).

The publication, not surprisingly, greatly upset the senior members and
officers of the Council. They were keen to point out that other lay members
had joined in a letter to the press disassociating themselves from her work
(not all lay members were signatories). The Council's response, published
in the *Lancet*, was long and detailed, to the point of nit-picking one might
say, drawing attention to many alleged inaccuracies; many of these were
challenged in the *Lancet* by Health Rights, her publishers. Her tone was
undoubtedly abrasive and there were some errors in her account, no one
can fully avoid such, especially when generalizing. The crucial point,
however, is that Jean Robinson was expressing the perceptions and experience of a world which is not inhabited by and is alien to the elite medical
world which dominates the GMC. The official reply exhibited the very
defensiveness which had in the first place led her to publish as she did and
which she believes is what has destroyed public confidence in the
profession.

What I have called the patients' revolt is only partially that, but there is
a sense in which if the 1970s was the decade of the profession, the 1980s
was the decade of the patient, especially of the patient seen as consumer.
The revolt came from different sources: from organized and disillusioned
patients who combined to improve care or gain or enforce rights, and from
a right radical government determined to break any kind of monopoly
power, whether of manual workers or of professionals. Strange bedfellows
and uneasy allies sometimes, for some of the patients' pressure groups
believe in the importance of a collective approach to health care as opposed
to a market approach. Yet they at last found ministerial allies in a right
radical government.

The patients' revolt was not perhaps so organized as the professional
revolt of the late 1960s and early 1970s—Jean Robinson has not quite
emerged as a Michael O'Donnell of the patients, but she has gone some
way towards it. Since the lay members are not elected, there can be no
strict parallel. But we do know the Privy Council reappointed Jean
Robinson after her book was published.

Whether those involved had intended it or not, lay control of the Council
would presumably have been the outcome had the revolution been as successful as was the professional revolution. In that upheaval elected

members were granted a majority in the GMC and the powers of the Council (and thus of the profession) were strengthened. But that was the culmination of a struggle which had begun with the GMC itself in the mid-nineteenth century. The patients' revolt only really began in the mid-twentieth century. Nevertheless, the conjunction of the patients' pressure groups and the Thatcher government undoubtedly clipped the wings of the medical profession as never before.

PART 5

FIT FOR THE TWENTY-FIRST CENTURY?

14

Profession before Public

The GMC needs reform

The accumulated evidence suggests that the GMC needs reform because it is not satisfactorily fulfilling its obligations to the state, namely that on behalf of the profession it will ensure that patients and potential patients may consult with trust the practitioners who are registered with it. It has not yet succeeded in renegotiating the education and training of doctors to fit the conditions of medicine of the late twentieth century. It has never really ensured the continued competence of registered practitioners. All the evidence suggests that when I served on the Council, and in the years before that, the Council had on balance resolved the many tensions it faced in regulating the profession in favour of the profession rather than the public. Now at the outset of the 1990s it is seriously attempting to deal with continuing competence to practise and, since its powers were increased in 1978, the education committee has been working towards the reform of education.

Despite these limitations of the GMC and the bodies it works through, the ethical standards of UK-doctors rank high world-wide. On the whole they have kept the service ethic to the fore and have not been readily corrupted. The profession—medical trade unions and prestigious educational bodies alike—has understood that it needs to continue to offer high-quality service if it is to retain its privileged position in the market. The GMC has been one—the crucial statutory one—among the many medical institutions which encouraged that outcome, albeit the GMC often appears to follow rather than to lead.

Nevertheless the Council has tended to favour the profession more than the public. This tendency was reinforced after the professional revolt of the 1960s, when the need to restore its legitimacy and the unity of the profession was paramount. Maintaining professional self-regulation, keeping the lay influence as low as possible, giving more voice to doctors hitherto unrepresented, were some of the methods used. The Merrison committee was instructed not to examine professional self-regulation so the committee did not enquire whether self-regulation did, in practice, work adequately in the public interest, or, if it was found wanting, whether modification was possible. Consequently, nothing in the Merrison Report operated as a check on the tendency to pay more attention to the profession than the people.

How the present situation has arisen

It is important to understand whether this tendency is built in to the very nature of professional self-regulation. For if it is, other regulatory modes must be found. How then has the present unsatisfactory situation arisen?

Its roots lie in the history summarized in Chapter 3. Frankly, the GMC was started to ensure the primacy of what was then allopathy over all the many other kinds of healing that abounded in the mid-nineteenth century. Historically, it has been modified largely to maintain the unity of the profession, from the addition in 1886 of elected representatives (so GPs could have a voice) to ceding a majority of the seats to those representatives in 1978. Other changes have followed the acquisition of further medical knowledge, the increased divisions in medical labour and the changing circumstances in which medicine is practised.

In 1858 the GMC was effectively a gentleman's club. Its promise that the public could trust those it registered amounted to ensuring that there were no 'bounders' in the medical fraternity [*sic*] who would do dastardly things such as no gentleman would do—or permit himself to be found doing. In the mid-nineteenth century committing adultery was a prime example of such inappropriate behaviour, as was making sexual advances to a patient or getting divorced. Committing murder was also not on. Discipline, then, was rather like black-balling club members, but ordinarily those black-balled were members of the profession at large, not of the GMC.

When I joined the Council in the mid-1970s it still had some of that air of a gentleman's club about it. One felt change was accepted reluctantly and that tradition dominated. It was really a place for white men for whom good food and drink was provided as a proper accompaniment to the serious work which was undertaken. The few women were tolerated and were treated very civilly (albeit their toilets were in basement or attic), but the ethos was male. There was no overt sexism or racism but a quiet acceptance of the superiority of white men and of the rightness of the established social order. Most members were quite unconscious of this ethos, so little had it then been challenged. I suppose I played a role which must have been irritating to many members of constantly drawing their attention to the ethos. Life on the Council was not entirely nineteenth century, of course; the founding fathers would have felt out of place in a number of ways. But given their pervasive legacy, they would have felt happier there than in many parts of the outside world.

The brotherhood of equals

The discipline which the profession accepted to ensure public and state recognition rested very heavily on a strong sense of brotherhood [sic] which was instilled in the course of medical education: pride in medicine, pride in one's particular medical school—loyalty is of the essence. Medical practitioners claimed, and claim, the uniqueness of their body of knowledge and set of skills; only they have this knowledge. To put it in technical terms, the profession is cognitively exclusive. It also sees itself as a community of equals. Registration makes all doctors of equal worth, whatever branch of medicine they practise in and whatever the material differences between them. This equality, however fictional it might be, given the numerous pecking orders within medicine, greatly helps to sustain the unity of the profession. It helps also to sustain the long hierarchical ladder to be climbed to reach registration and onwards to specialist status.

The strong sense of community, of solidarity, goes quite a long way to explain why there is such reluctance to strike practitioners off the register. Where a person has behaved quite outrageously, then there is no compunction. For the good name of the profession (as well as for the safety of the patients) they must go. But few cases are outrageous in medical eyes. If not outrageous, the reluctance to punish is manifest.

Reluctance is reinforced because 'it could happen to any of us'; 'if you, lay person, understood the conditions of practice you would know that there but for the grace of God...'. Justice should always be tempered with mercy, but only after the risks for patients have been well assessed. The patient also has a point of view: faced with a practitioner charged before the disciplinary committee the lay member can just as well say: 'In that surgery, clinic, hospital bed, might I, but for the grace of God, have been'. With a lay minority, those understandings cannot always be expressed and do not carry the weight of the shared practice experience. When the disciplinary committee is have ring about a decision, a firm lay statement 'I think that person is a danger to the public' may well tip the balance. Now there is more than one lay person at each disciplinary sitting it may be such statements can be more easily made, but the dominant ethos remains medical.

Keep the sheep in the fold

A concomitant of this strong sense of belonging to a unique and honourable profession is a great reluctance to see any member leave the fold. One might hear the disciplinary committee in effect say to a doctor 'You would be better off in another branch of medicine', or even 'You should only practise in the following branches of medicine' (indeed that might be a condition of continued registration). But one never heard 'Friend, we think you've strayed into the wrong profession, why don't you go away and retrain for something quite different?'. Members of Council are aware that some practitioners have been registered who were never or are not now suited to medical tasks. However, they have dealt with the problem by advising universities to pay more attention to the selection of students, a recurring theme, and to spotting early in their studies any misfits who may have unwisely been admitted to medical school. But once people are initiated, so to say, i.e. they have been accepted onto the register, every possible effort is made to keep them and return them to the fold if they do have to be suspended temporarily.

The importance of status

The value placed on the collectivity of medical practitioners is expressed in other ways as well. For the profession as a whole, as for other occupations which claim to be professions, collective status clearly matters a great deal (Macdonald, 1989). I have mentioned striving for honours. Historically, the GMC was an important part of the collective upward mobility of the medical profession and of the process of making it quite plain that physicians and surgeons were certainly not 'in trade'. Older members joked about that in the 1970s and 1980s, retelling stories of the days when, making a house call, one still risked being shown to the tradesman's entrance. In 1976—and no doubt still in 1990—status still mattered a good deal and was expressed in dress and demeanour. Members were proud of the honours they received from the Queen and hopeful that even higher honours might come their way. Other, lesser members basked in the reflected glory as their most outstanding colleagues were first knighted and then elevated to the peerage. For most this attachment to honours has not changed. Status striving motivates many.

Striving for high collective status is also expressed in the conspicuous consumption, elegance, ornateness, and waste of space which has gone into major professional buildings since the late eighteenth century. On all Macdonald's measures of these factors medical buildings score high. Professional members are prepared to put large sums of money into their buildings and to touch others for grants and subventions. Elegant though it is, the GMC building does not rate high compared with the Royal College of Physicians or the recently refurbished Royal Society of Medicine—a comment perhaps on the feelings of the profession about this statutory regulator, albeit it is their own. But nevertheless it has to be acceptable to people who frequent those more luxurious medical buildings. Collectively and individually doctors have come a long way: they have much to lose.

Guarding the portals

To maintain the standing of the profession, it is clearly important that the technical competence of new entrants should be assured. There is an associated wish that those admitted should be a credit to the profession in a social as well as a technical sense. With this goes a reluctance to admit to the fold any persons who do not fit or who in some way might 'let the side down'. This has less to do with technical competence than with their social acceptability as members of this exclusive collectivity.

Women were admitted to medicine most reluctantly and then, until the Todd Report, kept in a small minority by the use of a quota system in the admission of medical students (10% at University College, London, for example). Consequently one could be certain that those woman doctors who had qualified 20 years ago would be well above average ability and attainment. Yet few women were appointed to senior posts in the medical schools: it was taken for granted that a woman would not have a career such as a man might have. Women who did gain advancement in practice or academe found that they less often received merit awards, although men of similar status were preferred in that way. Furthermore, men as well as women were not aware that this was happening.

Discussion about the employment of women doctors revolved around the need for part-time appointments because of women's domestic responsibilities. The notion, increasingly a topic of popular discussion from the early 1970s onwards, that men might share the housework and child care, was never entertained in the Council—not even jokingly—in my earshot, or I guess out of it. The effect of medical education on the small minority of women who were admitted were to turn most of them in some respect into 'honorary males', albeit they were expected to retain their particular status as women in terms of sex, reproduction and domesticity. Thus socialized, the majority accepted their lot, colluded in the arrangements made and claimed they did not experience discrimination. The medical profession has a high suicide rate compared with other occupations, but that of women doctors is much higher than that of men. How far may this be a consequence of the personal conflicts engendered in them by the institutionalized male dominance?

With around half of the medical students and recent graduates of the last ten years now being women, this pattern must change. Women students and women junior hospital doctors now constitute a 'critical mass' and so can support each other and retain their identity as women. Change will be slow, as it always is in any time or place where the ceding or sharing of power is in question. The change have not yet worked through to the elite level of medicine and only in the last five year have they even begun to be reflected in the Council. For a member to mention that the GMC might be sexist and racist as Alison McCallum, newly elected Council member, recently did in the annual report (McCallum, 1989) is a change indeed. She perhaps got away with it because of her enthusiastic support for self-regulation.

The non-white

A similar restrictive process of reluctance to admit to full membership those who might not fit has operated—and still does—in the case of non-Caucasian doctors. The multi-cultural, multi-racial nature of modern British society is not reflected in the Council, although it lost its all-white face over ten years ago. The Council is not alone among British elites in being slow to admit the non-white. Nor is multi-ethnicity reflected very much in other prestigious places where doctors congregate.

Because of the nature of medicine and also of its chauvinism, a few non-white people educated in a UK medical school have for many years been accepted. They could be treated as honorary whites, as there were few enough of them (Lord Pitt is one who comes readily to mind). A few, properly educated as gentlemen, could be relied on not to rock the boat. To institute a colour bar as such has never been a British way.

It was when the large number of overseas doctors threatened to change the face (and thus, it was thought, the character) of UK medicine that restrictions became tighter. There were real problems of language and of the thoroughness of training and its appropriateness for British circumstances. The Council had been at fault in not being sufficiently careful about the standards of entry to the temporary register in the first place. What is really telling, however, is the total absence of any purpose-built training programmes for the in-comers whose labour the NHS so badly needed.

Induction programmes could have been initiated from a variety of places in the medical establishment or by the civil service. Their aim would have been to ensure that the in-coming doctors from the New Commonwealth and elsewhere understood what might be expected of them: in terms of language, of culture (the different gender order, for example), of the pathologies they might encounter most frequently, how the NHS worked and what UK postgraduate education was all about. However, the regulatory action taken was restrictive not educative. This is what makes one feel that the perceived inappropriateness of an influx of non-whites was a factor in the way in which overseas doctors have been treated. Only now, when there is an adequate supply of UK-qualified doctors, and tight immigration controls are in place, is there talk of one register. Hitherto for regulatory purposes 'overseas doctors' have been dealt with as a separate species. Like women, overseas doctors were often invited to sit at high table with the president during lunches taken between sessions: civilly treated, well looked after, but kept in their place, in fact gently and unobtrusively patronized.

Other healing modes

The establishment of the GMC gives a partial monopoly to biomedicine over all other healing modes. The GMC has in the past been quite restrictive about co-operation between registered practitioners and complementary or alternative practitioners. Generally speaking, registered practitioners may now refer to complementary practitioners so long as they keep ultimate oversight of and responsibility for the patient. There is no sense of co-operation at the elite level, although an increasing number of registered practitioners nowadays work with, for example, acupuncturists, homeopaths or osteopaths, or have learned some of their skills for themselves. Given the history of registration this stance is hardly surprising. The restrictiveness extends, however, to other health care professionals who are accepted as collaborators within the biomedical framework.

Other health care professions

The tight boundary which medicine has drawn round itself excludes other health care professions, but sets each in a clearly subordinate position to medicine. Each has struggled in various ways against this imposition (see, for example, Larkin, 1983). Medicine has remained intransigent. If a member of another profession, nursing, for example, or physiotherapy, with training and experience behind her or him, wishes to retrain to be a doctor, there is no way that the medical school takes any account of their previous knowledge, training and experience; they must tare the full complement of courses just as if they had come directly from school.

Insisting on a dominant position in the health care division of labour, historically having a large representation in the regulatory machinery of other health care professions, taking seats as of right on their boards of control, organized medicine has made no attempt to establish a reciprocal relationship with those other health professions. It was not until 1979 that a nurse sat on the GMC: she was appointed by the Queen in Privy Council as a lay member. In the present Council there is again a nurse and also a pharmacist—both 'lay' members. In the discussions preceding the 1978 Act no notice was taken of my suggestion that there should be seats for the other health care professions on Council allocated as of right. Anyone who is not a trained and registered practitioner is by definition 'lay' in medical eyes.

Yet the days of the one-to-one doctor–patient relationship are long over. Medicine is now a highly complex matter: a typical hospital treatment involves not only a number of doctors, nurses and others, but also non-medical personnel, technicians and the like, as well as the non-medical managers and executive staff who co-ordinate and run the service. In practice the profession no longer stands alone. This is even true in most modern general practice where the notion of a one-to-one relationship has more social reality, but even here the GP's work is backed not only by the surgery staff, but also by services, e.g. pathology laboratories, provided elsewhere.

Different personnel have the competence to understand and resolve each of the many facets of patient treatment. In health education, as in the establishment of appropriate conduct, medicine is unwise to ignore the contribution of other health care personnel. Yet the structure of the Council does not reflect the realities of the contemporary health scene.

Patients and potential patients

The boundary around organized medicine also excludes the patient and the patient's knowledge and experience from most aspects of medical decision making. Patients (more fashionably referred to nowadays as consumers) have a small place in the GMC, and no voice at all in the royal colleges and postgraduate medical education councils. Even in the universities, where the medical school is part of a much larger and predominantly 'lay' organization, medical schools are accorded remarkable amounts of autonomy, autonomy of a kind not accorded to other faculties. They have gained power on the basis of their claims to a monopoly of knowledge.

For the future

At what level and in what way other health care professionals, patients and potential patients should join with registered medical practitioners in the regulation of medicine, I shall discuss later. It is clear, however, that on a number of counts the GMC is not well poised to handle the regulatory problems of the 1990s. Reform is needed.

Not only the GMC: the Council in context

The array of regulatory procedures

In order to see what needs doing if the public are to be able to put reasonable trust in their practitioners, it is necessary to look at the contemporary context in which the GMC works. The first thing to note is the remarkable array in present-day Britain of procedures designed to regulate the profession in one way or another (see Stacey, 1991). The procedures may be divided into four types:

1. Professional, based on self-regulation;
2. NHS, of discipline and to handle complaints;
3. Parliamentary;
4. Legal.

These multiple modes of regulation have two main roots. The first lies in the concept of profession and professional self-regulation developed in the nineteenth century to succeed the more guild-like concept of the royal colleges and societies. Here the GMC is the crucial statutory body. The second root lies with the state: the increasing responsibilities felt by governments to ensure the provision of adequate medical care for their citizens.

The profession

One aspect of the professional mode, the GMC, is the subject of this book. Reference has also been made to the royal colleges, the faculties and the universities which continue to play important regulatory roles, as does the BMA which, while essentially being a trade union, does seek to enhance professional standards of practice and behaviour, and the defence societies, although Crown indemnity is now bound to alter their role. These bodies provide much of the immediate context in which the Council works. Medical audit is a rather different mode of self-regulation which has gained in significance in recent years.

Medical audit

Medical audit, under a variety of names, has been around for a long time, particularly in the USA. It differs from other sorts of collegial enquiry into medical practice, for example, 'grand rounds' or other forms of staff meeting and discussion, because of its systematic nature (the regularity of meetings, the use of numerate records and analyses) and the definitive inclusion of patient outcome. Other forms of collegial enquiry have tended to stress process rather than outcome.

In the UK, the Confidential Enquiry into Maternal Death set up in the 1930s by the Royal College of Obstetrics and Gynaecology (RCOG) is probably the earliest systematic peer review of outcome in clinical practice. The Association of Anaesthetists of Great Britain have commissioned three enquiries into anaesthetic deaths since the 1950s. There have been various enquiries into surgical performance and outcome, but nothing on the scale of the work of the anaesthetists or the RCOG. The Confidential Enquiry into Perioperative Deaths (CEPOD), covering anaesthesia and surgery, is a recent development aimed at filling this gap. This covered three regions only and has now been succeeded by the National Confidential Enquiry into Perioperative Deaths (NCEPOD). There have also been audits in the medical arena, but the examples, although important, have been somewhat scattered. The working party reports of the Royal College of General Practitioners (1985) are now setting the standards for audit in primary care.

Nevertheless, medical audit has not hitherto been widely, systematically or continuously applied to the process and outcomes of treatment. It now seems likely to be taken a great deal more seriously since its importance was underlined in the government's white paper *Working for Patients*, published in January 1989 (HMS0, 1989a). Two months later, a report from the Royal College of Physicians of London not only came out in favour of audit, but also made it clear that the College may withhold approval for hospital training posts if adequate medical audit meetings are not conducted.

The College stresses the equivalent importance in audit of structure (e.g. the quantity and type of resources), process (what was done to the patient), and outcome (in terms such as duration of survival, quality of life, residual disability). It insists that the cycle of audit, which includes standard setting, observing and comparing practice against standards, and implementing change, should always be completed.

Medical practitioners see medical audit as an essentially profession-led activity. They draw a clear distinction between clinical audit to improve patient care and managerial audit aimed at reducing costs; they wish to see these two activities kept separate.

The state

While medical audit had been started many years before the state began to press strongly for it, this history clearly demonstrates that the recent increased encouragement to audit is state inspired. It is another example of the profession tardily taking steps in an attempt to retain control of its working conditions through the medium of professional self-regulation.

The state's activities have a variety of aims, generally only secondarily concerned with the regulation of the profession as such. The state's interest lies with the health of the nation's people, closely associated as that is with the maintenance of social order; from this derives its concern with the provision and control of medical services. It also has the ultimate responsibility for the expenditure of public money.

The state's involvement has grown along with the immense development of medicine since the mid-nineteenth century—in scientific knowledge, in technology, in power to heal and in the damage medicine can do when misused or mistakenly used. To accommodate this expansion, the number of registered medical practitioners which the GMC has to control has increased four-fold since the 1930s. Medicine has pervaded very many more areas of the life of the nation and its people than the founding fathers of the GMC are likely ever to have imagined—so many more aspects of life are nowadays medicalized. As well as increased state involvement this medicalization process has meant that ordinary people nowadays think of health and illness in terms which are more like those of medical practitioners than the folk tales of yore—although important differences remain. Economic and social developments in the same period have also increased the standard of life, health, and level of education of ordinary people a great deal. Medical knowledge is not quite so esoteric any more. Withall, the relationships between the public and medicine and between patient and practitioner have been transformed.

The establishment by the state of the NHS, in which the great majority of doctors have worked for the past 40 years, has itself accelerated the expansion of medicine. It has made an important indirect contribution to professional regulation. The principle of a service free at the point of delivery has encouraged high ethical standards among UK doctors because that arrangement makes it possible for practitioners to offer the most appropriate treatment for a patient without consideration of who the patient is and their ability to pay. The temptation to overtreat inherent in fee-for-service or for-profit medicine is thus avoided.

The NHS has also contributed to the regulation of the profession in other ways, increasing the state's direct involvement in medical regulation through its own disciplinary and complaints procedures. The interest of the state in medical practitioners working for the NHS is different from its interest in the regulation of the profession as such—which it ceded in 1858 to the GMC—and has led to a different set of regulatory procedures.

Because of the different employment arrangements for hospital doctors and GPs, their mode of regulation within the NHS has been, and remains, different. With regard to those in NHS hospital practice, the Ministry of Health (as it then was) initially thought that the mode of accountability which applied to civil servants would be appropriate, since doctors are employed in hospitals on a salary basis. Later it became obvious that the nature of hospital medicine was such that purpose-built arrangements would be needed. Consequently, we now have two procedures: the disciplinary proceedings for medical staffs (under HM(61)112) and the complaints machinery for aggrieved patients or their representatives (HC(88)37). The latter is a relative latecomer, arriving ten years after the

Davies Committee on Hospital Complaints Procedures (Davies, 1973) had indicated machinery was necessary. The delay was on the medical side, coming particularly from the Royal College of Physicians.

With regard to GPs—and others like them who work as independent practitioners under contract to the state—the state's concern, which dates back to the National Health Insurance Act 1911, is that they fulfil their contracts. These practitioners are answerable for doing properly what they have contracted to do, but, in this context, answerable for that only. Any accountability to the state for the treatment, non-treatment or mistreatment of patients emerges as a secondary consequence of the requirement to fulfil the contracts. Like all others, family practitioners are also accountable to the GMC for their proper professional conduct and as citizens to the civil courts.

Parliamentary procedures

As an administrative apparatus the NHS is accountable to Parliament through its Board and the Department of Health. In terms of administrative justice the NHS and its staffs are also answerable to the Health Service Commissioner (HSC)—the Ombudsman. The HSC, however, has no jurisdiction over clinical matters; these, in consequence of the still upheld doctrine of clinical autonomy (of which more anon), are subject only to peer review. For junior doctors this means to their consultant in charge, and for the fully qualified either to peers in some form of medical audit or to the GMC if allegations of serious professional misconduct are involved. Medical practitioners may be held accountable to the HSC for maladministration in their NHS work, but not for their clinical decisions or actions. Parliamentary select committees (Public Accounts and Social Services) also hold a watching brief on behalf of the state.

Legal

All practitioners are subject, as are the rest of us, to the civil and criminal courts. The importance of the law with regard to medicine lies in the redress it may be able to offer to aggrieved patients. Patients or their representatives may have recourse to the law in order to establish 'the principle of respect for established legal rights or claims of the patient ... one of which is his [sic] power of determination' (Kennedy, 1983, p. 172). Cases may be brought to establish medical accountability to the patient. One reason is to gain compensation for a harm that the patient has suffered. Here the law can only act where negligence has been proved. In this procedure two goals are confused: pecuniary compensation for victims of medical negligence and medical accountability in the interest of that patient and patients at large.

The regulation of doctors in private practice

Those in independent private practice are answerable, as are all practitioners, to their individual patients for the treatment they give them and to the GMC for their professional conduct. Otherwise they are regulated only by the law. Those employed by a private firm or hospital are also formally accountable to their employing authority according to the contracts they have accepted, within the limits which law, custom and practice may bestow by virtue of their professional membership. Unless serious professional misconduct is involved, in which case a complaint may be made to the GMC, patients in private practice have no procedures available to them except legal ones.

An unsatisfactory array of regulatory procedures

None of the procedures taken singly nor the total array is felt to be altogether satisfactory. Discontent is felt (albeit for different reasons) by everybody who becomes involved one way or another with medical accountability, be they practitioners in the medical or associated professions, patients or their representatives, health service managers and administrators, policy makers, or governments.

In reviewing the four types of regulation of the profession, of its individual members and the profession itself as a collectivity, I have stressed how separate each of the four types is from the others. However, the distinctions associated with self-regulation, the NHS, Parliament and the law are less clear cut than one might expect from their various origins and intentions and the authority under which each is undertaken. The law appears to be the most independent but 'the law only ever requires the doctor to act in a way *other reasonable and informed doctors* judge to be proper'. In 'all other professions and walks of life, the standard of care by reference to which a person is judged is a matter for the court to determine. Expert evidence is *relevant but not determinative'* (Kennedy (1987), p. 59, first emphasis his, second emphasis mine; but see Havard (1989), pp. 12–13, on expert disagreements).

This principle is paramount throughout all the accountability procedures. Not only at law, but in any circumstance in which medical practitioners might be called to account, the profession has insisted that their peers should make the judgements. This insistence has been accepted at least since the GMC was established. It applies throughout the NHS. Professional self-regulation is clearly implicit in every form of medical accountability. It is the principle of essence.

Let me sum up the more important points about the array of regulatory procedures. First, if the procedures are not working well, the principle of self-regulation must itself be at least partly at fault. Second, the array is confusing to members of the profession as well as to the public; to the public because they are unclear where to go for what purpose; to practitioners because they may be arraigned for an alleged offence by a variety of authorities and for the same offence before more than one. This is so particularly for those working in the NHS: the law and the GMC may be involved but also one or other of the NHS regulatory procedures. On the other hand the regulation of doctors in private practice relies entirely on the GMC and the law. NHS doctors are thus subject to more regulation than those in private practice. There are also implications for patients: private patients have fewer channels open to them should they wish to complain about professional conduct.

Patients or their representatives who complain have one or both of two concerns in mind: the most common, to ensure that whatever they feel has gone wrong should not happen to anyone else; the second, and essential where earning power has been reduced or lifetime care is now necessary as a consequence of damage done, is to gain redress and compensation. A major problem is that these two goals are frequently confused in the present arrangements.

The law confuses pecuniary compensation for victims of medical negligence and medical accountability in the interest of that patient and patients at large. It is doubtful whether the law works well in either regard. The amount of compensation received is a lottery depending on the circumstances of the trial; where negligence is admitted the case is settled privately out of court and little deterrent effect may ensue. In general, there is no guarantee that anything will be done to rectify the situation for the future (Simanowitz, 1987, p. 118). Since 1982 increased attention has been drawn to these and other problems by Action for the Victims of Medical Accidents (AVMA).

15

False Gods and Collective Illusions

Reform of the GMC

Some of the changes which are needed are within the GMC itself: it is these that concern us here. However, what the GMC does has to be seen in the context of what other regulatory bodies do or propose to do. There are two risks here. One is reform which does little to improve the shape of the overall regulatory procedures. The other is the danger that the GMC may be tempted to wait on other developments. The evidence is that the GMC is aware that some initiatives now have to be taken.

The really important question, however, is whether the present GMC or a reformed GMC is able to do what needs to be done. Certainly the way the multiple procedures work out in practice could benefit from systematic review. It would seem unwise to go for piecemeal reform which might do no more than increase the confusing array. What is really at issue is whether professional self-regulation is appropriate in this day and age.

Is reform from within possible or likely?

In order that the public may be sure it can trust the registered practitioners who serve it, two lines of reform are needed. The first is reform of the GMC so that it performs its statutory tasks more satisfactorily. The second is the proper co-ordination of all the existing disciplinary and compensatory arrangements.

So far as the GMC is concerned a major question is whether reform can come from within or whether state action will have to be taken to achieve the necessary changes. Had I been asked ten or even five years ago whether that reform could be initiated from within the Council or would have to be imposed upon the profession, I would have said that I wished it could be undertaken by the profession, but I strongly doubted whether that was possible.

However, perhaps my doubts were unfounded. After a decade of 'consumer' activity is not the Council well on the way to reform from within? Some of the evidence suggests that: the new-style annual report introduced in 1989; the appointment of a public relations officer; the gradual increase in the number of lay members and making places available for them on a wider range of committees; the inclusion of a lay member in screening; the discussions of performance aimed at developing a new mechanism to ensure the continuing competence of practitioners. Change is certainly afoot.

Its leaders will tell you that it was Council which decided it needed more lay members, that Council itself saw the need to set the reforms in motion. My evidence is otherwise: Council leaders have been pushed and pushed and pushed again. They were pushed by the Privy Council which passed on messages from health ministers who did not share the faith of earlier administrations in professional self-regulation: ministers who were part of a government which was as at least as determined to break professional monopolies as it professed it was to break trade monopolies. It wanted to break up the old, smug, elite system in favour of a new and more fluid wealth-based social structure.

Council has also been pushed by its own lay member, Jean Robinson, and her supporters. Her views on consumerism (if not on other matters) are close to those of the present regime. Council has been encouraged by other members, medical and lay, albeit using somewhat different tactics from Jean Robinson, towards a variety of reforms.

During the 1980s Council might have liked some legislative changes in order to be able to conduct its business better. However, the evidence is that it avoided asking for this because the leadership was afraid that to start the legislative process would open the door for the inclusion of clauses reducing its powers. Council is now working hard to avoid a complete overhaul and to retain professional self-regulation; it is determined to show that this mode of regulation does work in the public interest and that it can reform itself adequately to do the job which the medical, social and political realities of the late twentieth century demand.

For my part I very much hope that the Council will be able to persuade itself and the rest of the profession of what is needed to achieve appropriate reform. Any labour force works better if its members are convinced of the need for the regulations under which they work. Occupational self-regulation is one way of trying to ensure that. The co-operative making of rules by the workers, their employers and other interested parties such as consumers (in this case patients and potential patients) is another.

Regulations imposed from above or outside lead to an alienation of the regulated which may make the regulations at best inefficient and at worst unworkable. In the case of medicine it is singularly important that the regulation works well. Lives are at stake. This is also true of many other occupations (those in charge of any form of public transport, for example, have lives in their hands). In addition, in medicine, indeed in all the health care professions and occupations, there are significant and important personal relationships included as well as the irreversibility, by their nature, of mistakes that may be made. The route of self-reform is, for these reasons alone, greatly to be preferred.

The Council has set out on this route. I am delighted. The question is can it go far enough? Will it be able to bring the other medical institutions—the BMA on the one hand and the royal colleges on the other—along with it? Will it be able to do that fast enough? Will it and they be able to stomach what is really needed—a reform of the Council which would change it beyond recognition, in which a great deal of the present power, so jealously held by Council and other bodies (colleges and universities particularly), would have to be ceded to others, in which, among other things, the lay voice was not only heard but understood and in which Council's work was clearly articulated to that of other bodies concerned with ensuring high standards of professional regulation?

Sharing power with others

A regulatory body has responsibility for maintaining standards and for setting them. It can, if it wishes and has the powers, offer guidance and leadership. How active it is, how much change it proposes, depends not only on powers, but on willingness to use them. The power, authority and influence of other medical organizations in a number of domains may encourage or impede changes the regulatory body may want. In the end a self-regulatory body can only be as good as the profession it regulates.

In disciplinary regulation difficulties may arise for the Council not only because of the intrinsic suspicion the regulated always have of the regulators, but also because of Council's remoteness from its rank and file. Difficulties deriving from this origin are most often expressed through the BMA or other trade-union-like groups of practitioners. Any solutions proposed, however, attract the interest of other medical organizations. In educational matters, while rank and file criticism is not uncommon, particularly from students and junior hospital doctors, the importance of the many other bodies becomes very obvious. The royal colleges in particular exercise a constraining influence, but so can the universities.

The universities

Initially the Council only had authority over basic medical education which was provided by the universities. It had no jurisdiction over specialist education or over continuing education. It was not until 1978 that it was required to promote high standards of medical education and co-ordinate all its stages. It still has no teeth with regard to any aspect of education except the basic.

This to some extent explains why progress in areas such as the pre-registration year has been so slow. Council has always exercised its powers quite delicately. For a long period it did not use its authority to visit or to inspect examinations except with regard to the new universities. Doubts cast on the sufficiency of the examinations by the royal colleges stung Council into action. No very tough line was taken officially with any of the universities, even where weakness was revealed. One could only hope that the universities would read between the lines of reports they received and that warning messages might be passed in a friendly and private manner; also that now inspections were being undertaken, their very existence would encourage raised standards. The Council's delight when the 1978 Act made it possible for them to appoint visitors to universities from among their own members rather than always having to appoint other members of the profession indicates how much Council members prefer to keep inspections with the home team and it perhaps indicates their dislike of the constraints they work under.

In everything it does the education committee and Council feel they must consult, and consult again, all those involved. It is apparently not enough that there are representatives of the colleges and universities on the education committee and the Council and that those bodies have already had opportunity to comment. They have to agree the final documents in many important cases. This makes progress slow and also gives the other medical bodies every opportunity to insert their preferred mode of action.

The royal colleges

Opposition from some of the royal colleges has held up the specialist register for over 20 years. The difficulties of trying to co-ordinate without teeth has meant that the relationship between the content of basic and specialist education still has not been satisfactorily worked out. The undergraduate curriculum remains overcrowded, the pre-registration year is still unsatisfactory. Nor, in the view of many, are the solutions when they are reached likely to make possible the readjustments which are needed. The shortfall between what the Council's advice indicates is a desirable medical education and what actually happens remains.

However, it is not only in educational matters that this slow consultation process takes place. Any serious change of policy or procedure has to be worked on carefully. Shortly after the Spearing Bill first came forward the then president, Sir John (now Lord) Walton, started personally going round all the relevant and powerful institutions to discuss what should be done to meet the mounting complaints which the bill expressed. Basically these were that bad practice was not being properly dealt with by the Council. The GMC then set up a working party which sat for two years. It is still working on the problem through a committee which advises the president. He speaks of introducing a new machinery to deal with the matters of competence which the Spearing Bill raised through examination of performance over time. In this interegnum Sir Robert Kilpatrick's utterances as president suggest that he is afraid to take a firm public line before agreement with all branches of the profession, within and without Council, is in sight.

The BMA

If the GMC has the royal colleges on one side, it has the BMA on the other. Ian Kennedy and others have suggested that the numbers of doctors disciplined has been restricted because the Council staff and members could not handle more cases. Fully adequate disciplinary procedures would undoubtedly cost more. Would practitioners be prepared to pay such increased costs so that the Council may remain independent? The question has surfaced sharply with the proposed increases in 1991. What view would the BMA take, representing as it does the material interests of the profession, but concerned as the leadership is with retaining independence? In the uprising of the 1960s and 1970s there were vociferous practitioners who did not want to pay more and who saw little point in independence.

It may not be simply a matter of staff size and thus of costs. It may be that the Council has been afraid of taking a tougher line, less because of the cost issue, than because it is afraid of losing its legitimacy with the profession if it disciplines practitioners more rigorously. Bringing forward a limited number of exemplary cases on those issues where the elite are agreed that discipline must be maintained rather than 'raking out and hauling up' all miscreants seems to have been the Council's practice hitherto.

But then the Council was not initially designed to be the apex of a complaints machinery . Member of the BMA from time to time make it plain in speeches or letters to the *BMJ* that they feel the GMC already disciplines much too much and irrationally. During the troubles around 1968 the BMA leaders, well interlocked with other parts of the elite, originally took a conservative line. As we saw in Chapter 4, a series of dissenting resolutions from the floor of the representative body was required to change that stance. It seems unlikely that the BMA would take a pro-patient stance. The BMA position alone is likely to restrict the Council's vision of its freedom of action.

The need to share power with other bodies and to keep the profession together seems to lead Council members into being quite gentle with fellow medical practitioners. Spending much time working closely with other sections of the medical elite also makes it harder for Council members to spend time learning to see things from the public's point of view.

The distance between the world of the GMC and the world outside

The distance between the world of the GMC and the world outside is much greater than most members of Council appreciate. By the world outside I mean the rank and file of ordinary doctors as well as patients and potential patients.

Rulers removed from reality

Not only medical governing bodies have this problem. People who are involved in the work of ruling (or regulating) come to view the world in distinctive ways (Smith, 1987, pp. 56–57). They share problems, experiences, concerns and interests in their committees and councils with others similarly placed (see, for example, Smith (1989j) on how large the GMC's *internal* problems loom to its staff and members). These experiences of the regulators are particular to them and markedly different from those of the people they are controlling—yes, albeit they are also medical practitioners. The continual focus on these everyday problems of governing can lead a ruling elite to become out of touch with its own rank and file as well as those it seeks to serve. This became very plain around 1968 when the profession revolted against the GMC. Lay as well as medical members can become removed from everyday reality. The lay, furthermore, have no constituencies to turn to, except for those who were nominees of community health councils and chose to use them as informal constituencies.

This mode of ruling works well as long as the majority remain silent. The elite's authority and power depends upon the silences of those who do not participate, who are outside the process. In the case of the practitioners this means that the registered practitioners accept the charges and constraints imposed on them by the GMC; in the case of the public it means that the complaining patients and their representatives accept without overt objection the kind of cases that are heard and the verdicts that are passed. There may come a time when the silences are broken: the profession broke silence around 1968. The patients became increasingly vociferous in the 1980s. In circumstances like these the legitimacy of the elite ruler is challenged.

The particular medical gap

In the case of the GMC the gap between the regulators and the public on behalf of whom they work has some distinctive features. Of the three characteristics of the profession—its unity, its service ethic and its exclusiveness—the last isolates the profession and leads to in-turningness and seeming arrogance. The claim of exclusive knowledge also creates a gap between practitioner and patient, a gap which is not well understood in the profession, being seen as a problem in the mode of communication. In reality much of the problem derives from different knowledge bases: the trained knowledge of the practitioner and the experiential knowledge of the patient and potential patient. Each rests on different premises and selects different aspects of the evidence as relevant for explanation from the other. Both approaches are valuable, relevant, meaningful and necessary for the proper evaluation of a conduct case as well as for a clinical case.

In writing about this gap I have often used an example derived from Priscilla Alderson (Alderson, 1988) who has shown how complex are the problems in ensuring informed parental consent to a child's proposed cardiac surgery, not least because the knowledge, which informs the cardiac team is of a different order and takes different factors into account from the knowledge which informs the parents. The latter includes an understanding of the meaning for their child and for themselves of the long-term sequel, should the outcome bring life, but also brain damage—how should the parents weigh this against the possibility of the child not having any long-term life at all?

One senior member rejected this example, saying it was something quite different from a case before the GMC. He implied that whatever distance there might be between aggrieved patients whose complaint had led to a GMC hearing and members of the committee hearing the case, it was of a different order from issues of informed consent and the distance in a treatment situation. Certainly the two examples have important variations in detail, but both come from the same fundamental differences between the two worlds, medical and lay. His comment reinforced my point that the meaning of an alleged misconduct is different for a patient (or patient's relative) and for a practitioner. The whole episode, or series of episodes, are seen differently by each. The differences derive from similar sources to those in the informed consent case. The run-up to the decision to operate offers quite different data to parents and practitioners; so does the run-up to a disciplinary hearing. In the latter case, the differences include elements of the done-to versus the doer and of the aggrieved versus the accused. But perhaps most importantly the understanding of the situation in one case derives from everyday experience of health, ill health and expected medical behaviour; in the other it is located in the conditions of medical work, the medical knowledge which motivates or should motivate action.

There is of course a level at which the best interests of the patients, taken as a whole, are also the best interests of the profession, taken as a whole. However, in particular cases and in practice differences emerge. The medical world has a reality to medical members which the patient world does not. I recall the case of the single-handed GP charged with prescribing drugs other than for bona fide treatment. In his defence it was argued that he had been threatened by an addict, that he was alone and could do no other than accede. No one thought to ask whether there was anybody in the waiting room from which help might have been summoned: 'no one' seemed to mean no other doctor, no nurse, no receptionist, no 'real' person, or at least no reliable person.

It is the custom of the Council, if business requiring outside personnel looks like having to be held over until the next day, to enquire whether any persons may be seriously inconvenienced and if so to try and accommodate them. On one occasion adjourning a disciplinary hearing meant that two elderly witness from afar, totally unaccustomed to London and intimidated, as most are, by the GMC procedures, had to stay unexpectedly overnight. Their well-being was not enquired after and their distress at being called at all was thereby increased. I noticed what was happening but too late to stop it. When I spoke to the president about it the next morning, he was greatly distressed that this should have happened. He had not realized; but he had been in the chair, making the enquiries about the implications of the adjournment. He had not meant those two to be treated as if they were not 'real people', as if their life and time was less important that that of solicitors, barristers or medical witnesses, but that was what had happened. Those who do not belong and do not have power somehow do not exist. The damage is not intended, but it is done nevertheless.

Bridging the gap

The gap is not totally unbridgeable, however. I have noted two sorts of bridge-building. One kind occurs when a doctor, usually young and without vast amounts of clout, has a disquieting experience with a relative.

The other is when doctors are motivated to take a new look at long-standing assumptions using systematic research evidence.

The *BMJ* printed an example of the first in 'Personal View' (Anon., 1989). The author's father died the day she or he graduated from medical school. The death occurred after what should have been a routine operation and apparently resulted from a lack of attention to the case initially by medical but also by nursing staff. And this despite the presence of the young graduate who was acutely aware that matters were not as they should be and who tried to get proper attention paid to the patient, her or his father. The happenings were 'unbelievable' but a 'painful reality'. The author concludes that greater accountability might have prevented this tragic death. Such 'unbelievable' happenings might well not be believed were it a 'lay' person presenting the evidence. The account would certainly be unlikely to be published in the *BMJ*. Indeed, until recently this medical account might well not have been published on the grounds that the account as given 'broke ranks'. Publishing the case helps to bridge the patient–practitioner divide—as well as revealing something badly wrong.

The second example relates to sexual relations between doctors and patients. In medical circles, and particularly when taking to lay people about sexual interference with their patients by doctors, the context of discussion has in the past rested heavily on the great risks that doctors run at the hands of their patients; tales are told of the 'siren' who comes into the surgery determined to have the practitioner lay her. This is a long-standing story; given that male doctors were heavily in the majority until recently and given also the generally heterosexual and patriarchal values of the society in which we live, it is not surprising that the tales are of female patients and male doctors. I have not yet heard a version which takes into account the increasing number of female doctors; they are mentioned when discussing guidelines or cases, but not in the tale-telling context. I have heard many varieties of the tale, but they are so essentially similar that one knows they partake of the qualities of a myth, a folk-tale, a story told, according to Malinowski, the anthropologist, as a charter for action.

Faced with this body of 'knowledge' and its mode of presentation, this lay woman has found it difficult to convey the knowledge of so very many women that minor, and sometimes not so minor, sexual advances or innuendo are not uncommonly made by male doctors to their female patients, patients who had come for nothing more than professional diagnosis and treatment. In their study of doctors and patients in Swansea, Stimson and Webb (1975) report that one of the GPs there was known to the patients as 'Doctor Undress' because of his propensity to have his female patients undress whatever their complaint was. (Another was known as 'Two-Minute Todd' because of his speed of working: there were other nicknames also, all pseudonyms for what the informants actually called them.) The existence of a 'Doctor Undress' was challenged by some critical readers. This was not the traditional tale of sexual relationships between doctors and patients, which showed the strength of most and excused the occasional lapse of a few.

Nigel Fisher and Thomas Fahy (Fisher and Fahy, 1990) have now opened up this discussion, commenting that the GMC has never done so. They suspect that the cases of sexual interference by doctors with their patients which come to the GMC represent the 'tip of an iceberg'. They use evidence derived from two American surveys: the first is of 1442 practising psychiatrists (a 26% response rate), in which 7% of male and 3% of female respondents (6.7% overall) acknowledged having had sexual contact with their own patients. In the second, 10% of psychiatrists, 18% of obstetricians, 13% of GPs and 12% of internists either confessed to or condoned erotic behaviour in the doctor–patient relationship. Fear of litigation has prompted the research and the action in the USA. A centre for victims of therapist abuse in Minnesota attracted 1500 victims in its first four years in operation. A Wisconsin psychiatrist (Palermo, 1990) elaborates on the special problems of psychotherapist–patient sex, providing further evidence of its not uncommon occurrence. Fisher and Fahy believe similar evidence would be found for the UK and conclude that the most important thing is for the profession to recognize that there is a serious problem.

In my terms Thomas and Fahy are saying that the myth which is supported by the tales of the sirens—the myth that the patients and not the doctors are to blame—is no longer of use to the profession; indeed the myth is disadvantageous to it as well as to the patients. I spoke of a myth or a folk-tale as a charter for action. The myth of the sinning patient and the upright but sorely tempted doctor prevents cases coming forward for adjudication. And should they come forward the strength of the myth prevents the practitioners who are considering the case from listening to the evidence objectively, for all women have become tarnished with the siren's brush. The action (unconsciously?) intended by the tale is to protect the professional male from exposure by female patient—or, suitably modified, the other way round.

This section began with a discussion of the gap in knowledge and understanding which exists between patient and practitioner, and thus between most members of the GMC and the public they are there to protect. These two examples show that from the side of the profession attempts can be made to close the gap in experience and knowledge. Its existence has first to be recognized. It is the recognition and articulation of a problem which is encouraging about the publication of these articles. The discussion of the sex myth has, however, also shown that some parts of the gap are created, albeit sometimes unconsciously, for the protection of the profession.

False gods and collective illusions

The Council has embarked on a number of important reforms. The cynical view would be that Council are only moving now because they are under pressure and they want to retain self-regulation: a respectable enough goal in itself. The more optimistic view is that leaders and members have now understood the need for radical reform and they intend to make professional self-regulation work better in the public as well as the professional interest. Maybe a good deal of encouragement from medical and lay members inside the Council and from outside sources was needed, but members now recognise that all has not been well, or at least is not acceptable. I think the latter is a real possibility.

I am inclined to think that in the past well-meaning members of the Council, and of the profession at large, have simply not understood that the Council has been doing a bad job in terms of what is expected of them by the public; nor do they yet really understand why that has been so. My view is that they are deluded by certain tenets about professionalism which were useful in the mid-nineteenth century but which now are no more than collective illusions which misguide rather than guide the profession. But an understanding that this is so is beginning to develop in a variety of medical quarters.

My conclusion is the result of working on a difficult research problem. The problem was to understand how it could be that essentially decent and well-meaning men (mostly men) of high ethical standards could operate a system which colluded in the maintenance of an out-dated educational system and served the public so ill in matters of discipline and competence. If both parts of this proposition are true, that the Council works badly in the public interest (and, as I believe, also in the professional interest) and that most members sincerely wish to do a good job, it can only mean that they have no idea what they are doing. I believe this may be true. If it is true, it may at least in part be because doctors cling to certain tenets of professionalism which blind them to the realities of contemporary medical practice.

Much of the thinking which guides the profession has been based on the notion of the one-to-one doctor–patient relationship. While there is still something in this notion, as we have seen, it is to some extent a myth in terms of the contemporary reality of medical practice. It was used successfully to fend off managerial control in 1974 as was noted in Chapter 2 where the crucial statement (DHSS, 1972, 1.18) was quoted in full. Reality, in the shape of problems (not least cost) created by modern complex medicine, has since overcome this myth and clinicians are now both involved in management and subject to management. They may dislike it, but most now accept that it has to be the case.

Closely associated with the one-to-one doctor–patient relationship is the doctrine of clinical autonomy—that only she or he who is in charge of the case may make decisions about it, that no one else is capable of offering judgement, and that only peers may comment on its rectitude should it be questioned. Sir Raymond Hoffenberg (1987) in his Rock Carling lecture said clinical freedom was 'of course, a chimera': personal, moral, ethical and even legal constraints on clinical decisions have always existed and properly been observed (p. ix). Hoffenberg further argued that the medical profession is mistaken in continuing to believe in this chimera as a guide to their actions. As an example he analysed critically the excited professional reaction to the limited drugs list (p. 29). The belief in clinical freedom is not only a chimera, but is one of the many collective 'subjective illusions' to which the profession clings and which are nowadays of little use to it.

There is also no need to cling to the special expert status whereby only doctors can determine what is right in medical matters. My experience suggests that, given interpretation of the medical language used and the inferences made from the data, non-medical persons are perfectly capable of coming to wise conclusions. Indeed, in the face of conflicting medical evidence, and medical cases are by no means open and shut as to the facts or their interpretation, a non-medical adjudication can be positively helpful.

Other kinds of myths exist to protect the profession and its members. We have seen that the myth that practitioners do not make sexual advances to their patients except when they encounter determined and seductive females is in the course of being exploded by systematic medical research.

It is also illusory to believe that the exclusiveness, so long cherished by the profession, is really of vital professional and personal importance. Indeed, as we have seen, it has particularly negative consequences in cutting members of the profession off from the people they serve and from others with whom they work. In an interesting analysis, Steve Watkins (1987), a public health doctor, has drawn attention to what a powerful and dominant profession medicine is—and this remains so despite the many attacks it has suffered in recent years. Yet, as he says, medicine as a profession and medical people as individuals constantly feel embattled and powerless. In his view, medicine, by its exclusiveness and its seeming arrogance, its refusal to share power with other professionals, other health workers, patients' groups or democratically elected representatives of the people, has itself created the very opposition it so much fears. But few medical practitioners understand this.

Medicine's main weapon against this hostile world, Watkins argues, is its absolute unity achieved by being depoliticized and highly conformist. The conformity is deep. The views which the profession holds are right because the profession holds them; professional norms are loyally followed. Yet, as Watkins asserts, the profession is fiercely independent:

> Doctors protest their independence and individuality but in fact this is a myth in which, in true conformity, they believe ... The medical profession is organised along the principle that once you have ensured that people conform loyally to the right ideas you can allow them a considerable degree of independence of action
>
> Watkins (1987), p. 21

To pursue Larson's (1977) insight which I have been using, medical practitioners share the subjective illusion; their training has ensured that they believe in the correctness of their cognitive exclusiveness.

Deviants are tolerated as eccentrics, thought of fondly, but not listened to. The really rebellious, however, are victimized; their career advancement blocked. This may not happen very often, but the knowledge that it can happen is enough to ensure the conformity of the majority (Watkins, 1987, p. 30). However, at the same time, and for the same reasons of maintaining the unity of the profession, incompetent doctors may be shielded. What is more, interlopers may sometimes be admitted and get away with it partly because of the very acceptance offered to the qualified. Who could imagine such a thing anyway?

Paper Mask

In my days on the disciplinary committee I sat on the case of a doctor who was charged with serious professional misconduct for posing as a doctor when he had no qualifications (see Chapter 11, pp. 144–145). While obviously potentially very serious that an untrained person should be able to get away with such a pretence, I found the case in many ways funny. My medical colleagues on the committee took it all terribly seriously; no way was there a twinkle in anyone's eye. Indeed, they took this case more seriously than many others I sat on, others which had distressed me much more, for example where a doctor, in independent practice, fully qualified and registered, was charged with serious professional misconduct when a death had resulted from his practice of medicine. The case of the pretender had, for the doctors on the committee, none of the mitigating features of a situation they recognized where each felt 'that disaster, but for the grace of God, could have happened to me'. They, after all, had done their six or seven years training and more besides.

There were two reasons why I found sitting on that case funny. First, the idea that a pretender could get away with it for a while is always good for a laugh. No serious damage was reported as having been done. All except the most prim of us must find a mischievous sense of fun is evoked when an intruder has managed to con so solemn (sometimes even pompous) and well-barricaded a body of people. The second reason was that we were in technical problems about disciplining the guy. A registered medical practitioner can be charged with serious professional misconduct; that indeed was the charge. However, how could one find someone guilty of serious professional misconduct and strike them off the register when they had never been on it in the first place? In the end we did just that.

Recently I went to see *Paper Mask* (director, Chris Morahan, GB, 1990), a film about a biology drop-out turned hospital porter who poses as a junior hospital doctor and gets away with it—at least until the end of the film and possibly indefinitely thereafter. He is 'the Great Pretender' of the film's theme song. I did not find the film funny, that mischievous humour was not evoked—there were amusing episodes of course, but overall I found the film upsetting.

I found it upsetting for many reasons. The hyper-realism of the accidents with much simulated and overly red blood, indeed the hyper-realism of the entire film in terms of make-up, angles of shots and so on, was typical of many modern films. The dominant lack of morality, not only in the main character, the Great Pretender himself, but also among more senior doctors, the corruptibility of the formerly upright sister, the failure to act of the one senior doctor who appeared to have high ethical standards, were all features typical of many contemporary films of the 'post-modern' period. My hopes that 'good' would prevail, that someone would blow the whistle in the interests of the patients, indeed in the interests of medicine itself, the sister (who had lost her job because of him), the caring and efficient senior perhaps, were too old-fashioned and doomed to be dashed.

This was not a film about someone sending up the system and having a good run for her or his money. No, it was a medical thriller but also an exposé of a rotten system, a system out of control, where personal self-interest or collective self-interest conspired to let the rogue get away with it in an escalation of tragedy. Tragedy for the senior consultant whose powers are failing, who had made 'mistakes' but who would not retire and was not pushed out but moved sideways. He it was who chaired the meeting which appointed the Great Pretender, failing hopelessly to interview properly and preventing others from doing so. His wife it was who was killed by the pretender in casualty in the course of reducing a coppis fracture. This doctor was ultimately responsible for his wife's death but not in the way he thought. He along with the court wrongly believed a badly maintained cuff was at fault (for which he was managerially responsible), so he shot himself. Tragedy for the sister who left a job and career, which she seemed to enjoy and be good at, to cover for her lover. Tragedy for the good guy, the hospital porter who turned up to retrain as a nurse—and who would have made such a good nurse—but in so doing stumbled upon his old mate in his new guise. He was relieved of his life in consequence.

But the Great Pretender moved on to a new appointment. His career continued because no one blew the whistle: doing so would hurt them or the system. The ethically minded and caring consultant hesitated to act because of the consequences for the hospital and medicine more widely if he did. Better to say nothing. The subjective illusions about how the profession should be run and which I have been arguing are today so totally inappropriate were one root of the problem.

This film (and indeed John Collee's book which he adapted for the film) is the most serious indictment of professional self-regulation I have ever seen, heard or read. It is a serious indictment not only because it was written by a doctor, an insider's account, but because it offers no hope for the future. This is not an account of a bad guy who gets away with too much because of weaknesses somewhere but is finally found out, probably at someone's considerable personal expense. It is an account of a system within which there seems to be no chance of the whistle being blown. So there is no morality and no hope.

It does not matter that there may never have been a case like the Great Pretender, or as bad as that, or that there may have been. What is crucial is that the book was written, the film was produced and in the genre that was used. Other similar films are made and books written. Many are on other topics than medicine. They express what Elizabeth Wilson (1990, p. 147) has called 'the ethical vacuum of the "postmodern" society'.

I believe this ethical vacuum has resulted from the failure of our society, specifically of its elite system, to live up to its claims of trustworthiness, and our inability so far to produce a viable alternative. We have lost faith in the scientists, the doctors and other professionals who were supposed to be the upright men [sic] of our society. Our overwhelming sense of powerlessness has also tarnished our faith in democracy. Trust is lost, so morality goes.

One could argue that Collee's exposé is an improvement on the old apologia which helped to retain the illusion that all really was well among the powerful—despite a few rogues whom we all knew about. In writing it John Collee broke ranks with the medical 'brotherhood'; he is unlikely to achieve advancement in the system; he has brought medicine into disrepute. As *Time Out* put it 'Just when you thought it was safe to go back in the hospital ...'. But to what point did he write this? Was there no other way? Perhaps not. Or none that would have made so much money? What happened to the service ethic? Or is Collee's way the only way to talk about our distress at the loss of trust?

The problem is not just one for medicine, it is a problem for the entire society. But because of its ethical basis, medicine is in a good position to take measures to restore social trust in itself and this could be an important beginning not only for medicine but also for the larger society.

16

Can Self-regulation Work?

The service ethic and the changes made

Although, as Watkins (1987) points out, many of the ethical rules have to do with restrictive practices, some are idealistic principles about dedication to patient care. They derive from the strong service ethic and, Watkins argues, are powerful motivators of idealistic behaviour which ensure that responsibility to the patient is stressed and confidentiality given the highest priority. He correctly points out that in oppressive regimes doctors have been imprisoned for refusing to break these ethical rules.

My evidence suggests that it is through the notion of dedication to good patient care that movement away from narrow professional interests can be, indeed is being, achieved. Some might say more cynically, perhaps, that if forces outside the GMC insist on such a move it is in those terms that the leadership can justify them to the profession. There have undoubtedly been changes. These have taken place in the areas of discipline, sick doctors, ethical guidance, education, and lay representation and involvement. How significant one judges these changes to be depends on what one thinks the GMC should be doing, what it is there for. I shall come to that presently. First, let me draw together the changes that have been made or are afoot.

Changes in the blue book

Analysis of changes over the last ten or 15 years in the blue pamphlet of guidance on professional ethics published by the GMC shows a trend away from narrow restrictive professionalism towards greater stress on good patient care. Comparing the blue pamphlet of 1987 with its predecessor of 1976, I concluded it was much different (Stacey, 1990). It still devoted a good deal of space to intra-professional ethics, issues such as canvassing and advertising, which had taken most of the space in 1976. However, in 1987 there was much more in it that was patient-oriented.

Specifically a number of issues to do with the confidentiality of the information which a doctor may have acquired about a patient had been developed, as had issues to do with standards of the medical care of patients. The extensive section on relations with the pharmaceutical industry should also be mentioned in this connection. These changes, my analysis suggests, came about in consequence of pressure from the media, from government and from other lay sources. However, that they are made at all derives from the recognized importance of ensuring good service to the patients.

Conflicts between 'brotherhood' and service

The conflict between the supposed interests of the profession and the profession's commitment to the best interests of the patient has its legacy in the guidelines. This emerged clearly in a dispute which arose between Jean Robinson and the Council over doctors' responsibility to each other versus their responsibility to their patients. In the development of the blue book over the last 15 years additions had been made which spelled out the limits of unconditional 'brotherhood'. Doctors were now permitted to disagree with the advice of others, and they might advise patients to seek treatment elsewhere without risking a charge of serious professional misconduct. Furthermore, in 1989 they were now required to

> inform an appropriate body about a professional colleague whose behaviour may have raised a question of serious professional misconduct, or whose fitness to practise may be seriously impaired by reason of physical or mental condition.
>
> GMC (1989), paragraph 67, p. 17

This was a far cry from the largely self-protective emphases of earlier guidelines.

These passages came in a section of the blue book called 'Disparagement of professional colleagues'. The section put the issue of complete loyalty and unity first:

> It is improper for a doctor to disparage, whether directly or by implication, the professional skill, knowledge, qualifications or services of any other doctor, irrespective of whether this may result in his [sic] own professional advantage, and such disparagement may raise a question of serious professional misconduct.
>
> GMC (1989), paragraph 65, p. 17

Jean Robinson argued that this paragraph should be expunged. She feared it took away from the force of the following paragraphs which stressed responsibility to the patients. The standards committee of the GMC did not then agree with her, although they discussed it fully and conceded she had a point. It seemed the emphasis on unity prevailed. That was what, ironically, protected the Great Pretender in the *Paper Mask*.

As I noted with regard to the Sharp and Sultan affair (Chapter 13), Raanon Gillon, editor of the *Journal of Medical Ethics*, opened a debate on this dispute in 1990, inviting contributions, not only on the straightforward question of whether that paragraph should be deleted, but on the much wider one of the responsibilities of individual practitioners and the profession as a whole to ensure by a variety of means that standards of medical practice remain high.

The response to this and the earlier criticisms made came during the November 1990 meeting of Council which led to a new edition of the blue book being published in February 1991. The heading of the relevant section has been changed from 'Disparagement of professional colleagues' to one headed 'Comment about professional colleagues' (GMC, 1991, p. 16, paragraphs 62–64).

The first paragraph (62) refers to the frequency with which doctors are asked to express views about their colleagues, whether in audit or peer review, writing a reference, when a patient seeks a second opinion, specialist advice or an alternative form of treatment. 'Honest comment', the paragraph concludes, 'is entirely acceptable in such circumstances, provided that it is carefully considered and can be justified, that it is offered in good faith and that it is intended to promote the best interests of patients.' Paragraph 63 then refers to a doctor's duty to inform appropriate authorities where a colleague's 'professional conduct or fitness to practise may be called into question or whose professional performance appears in some way to be deficient'.

Only in the third paragraph does the issue of loyalty to colleagues arise. Paragraph 64 reads:

> However, gratuitous and unsustainable comment which, whether directly or by implication, sets out to undermine trust in a professional colleague's knowledge or skills is unethical.
>
> GMC (1991), p. 16

Stricter discipline

There have also been changes in the disciplinary procedures. Unsatisfactory though many people still find them, there have been increased efforts to maintain standards and to do it fairly and humanely. It was Lord Cohen, as we saw in Chapter 3, who insisted that the Council become more active, including in disciplinary matters—this did not increase his popularity with the rank and file but earned him a great deal of respect among his peers. Since then the frequency of sittings has increased greatly; the number of lay members at any one sitting has been increased from one to two and a lay person included in the preliminary procedures.

The health committee

Perhaps the most important change was the introduction of the health committee which made it possible to separate the mad from the bad—or the sick from the wicked or incompetent. This is a much more humane approach in intra-professional terms. The independent, but linked, intro-duction of the welfare arrangements for sick doctors also increases the chances of help being obtained for them. These two developments are likely to improve medical safety from the patient point of view. We lack objective evidence to know how much difference these measures have made on the ground in terms of what needed to be done. The problem is we had no measures of how big was the iceberg whose tip, in cases coming to discipline, was all that previously could be seen.

Performance reviews

There will be change, as we have noted already, in the direction of ensuring the maintenance of competence, but that has not yet arrived, nor is the shape it may take entirely clear.

Slow progress in education

In education progress seems slow and this was admitted by Professor David Shaw, the chairman of the education committee in the 1989 *Annual Report*:

> The Medical Act 1978 sought to allow greater freedom in medical education than before. It paved the way for a liberation of the curriculum ... But the shackles have not loosened in any significant way.
>
> Shaw (1989), p. 17

So the committee, ten years later, will try again. There have been advances towards specialist registration, so far on a voluntary basis.

Perhaps the most movement (small though it may be in terms of what has to be done) has come on those fronts where the service ethic is most directly involved. This is encouraging.

Changes not yet sufficient

When Watkins wrote in 1987 he saw the GMC as having significance beyond its relatively limited statutory functions because of two important roles it plays in the maintenance of the status of the profession. The first is to ensure, through a system of restricting the profession to those properly qualified and expelling any who do not conform to the ethical standards laid down, that the profession is seen as a body of highly qualified, independent servants of the public. The second is to ensure that doctors are socialized into the thought processes and norms of behaviour of the profession (Watkins, 1987, p. 24). This process takes place in the medical schools and the associated hospitals, but it is the GMC which makes the education compulsory. What I think Watkins is referring to are the roles which I have perceived as crucial for the GMC, namely maintaining the unity of the profession and its national standing. He would not argue that the GMC fulfilled all aspects of these functions itself, but that its role as the statutory body was crucial. Certainly when I served on the Council these pro-professional enterprises appeared high on the agenda. Despite the changes which I have outlined, the GMC had not by 1987, according to the Watkins analysis, fundamentally changed its role.

Richard Smith, after undertaking extensive interviews with a wide range of people wrote, a series of nine articles on the GMC in the *BMJ* (1989b–j). He exposed the criticism and discontent with the GMC felt by many. His conclusions were highly critical of every aspect of its work. He examined the size and nature of the secretariat upon which the GMC depends (something which I did not include in my study) and was sceptical concerning the absence of professional skills among both members and staff on a number of issues, notably education. As to the membership, he felt perhaps that there was too much for part-time members to do.

In their turn his articles drew a good deal of criticism from those who felt that the GMC was much misunderstood and was doing a better job than he suggested—see, for example, the vehement letter signed by David Bolt, Ronald Robertson, David Innes William, John Walton and Henry Yellowlees, all of whom then were or had been members of the GMC and four of whom were also present or past presidents of the BMA (*BMJ*, 1989). Smith's criticisms, of education, of the maintenance of competence, of the failure of the Council properly to be able to take account of public opinion, of the mysterious way in which Council operates, all make sense to me. They chime with my evidence. Change, however, is on the way.

What the GMC proposes to do

The GMC is well aware that further reforms are necessary if it is to retain any legitimacy with the profession or with the public and government. It is possible, as Richard Smith pointed out, that the GMC might be swept away altogether (Smith, 1989b) if it does not meet it critics. This it is trying to do and will put forward proposals for legislation to that end. Most members are aware that the GMC must be modified to meet the more serious of the complaints that are currently made against it. Of these the failure to stimulate revision of the undergraduate curriculum, the failure to ensure continuing competence and the continued existence of two modes of registration of overseas doctors the GMC recognizes as the most serious. They were referred to by the president both in his response to the *BMJ* articles (Kilpatrick, 1989) and in the *GMC Annual Report for 1989*, (p. 2).

Discipline

With regard to disciplinary matters, as the president put it:

> As far as the disciplinary work of the Council is concerned we have been considering two major issues: the involvement of a lay member in the initial screening of complaints and a new procedure for reviewing doctors' professional performance as an issue separate from serious professional misconduct. This performance review would involve an assessment of a doctor's clinical competence and professional attitudes which would by no means be a 'lesser charge' than serious professional misconduct. The setting up of such a procedure will be a long and complex task, one which a working group has already begun, involving detailed discussion with a wide variety of interested parties, including professional and public organizations.
>
> *GMC Annual Report for 1989*, p. 2

These proposals undoubtedly represent a major advance in Council's thinking. Whether '*a* lay member' is an adequate addition to the team of medical screeners remains doubtful, given the heavily dominant medical ethos. However, this is a great advance on the situation when I first joined the Council. Then it was impossible to get any meaningful information at all about the screening process and a general impression was cast of the high proportion of the 'dotty' who complained. 'If you saw the letters, Margaret, you would realize they were definitely disturbed.' Perhaps, but I did not see them, nor did others, except the president and the section of the registrar's office which dealt with them. The more times I heard that story the more I became convinced it was yet another traditional tale, told this time with the purpose of retaining control and the *status quo*. What better than to dismiss most of the complainants as mad, sight unseen?

As to the issue of performance, the discussion began with Spearing's suggestion that there should be a conduct charge of lesser gravity than serious professional misconduct. The Council were and are implacably opposed to two standards of conduct. The whole matter was really one of the way in which the Council went about ensuring the continued competence of registered practitioners. What is now being discussed is not outcome but performance. Patients are interested in outcome; the profession is interested in process. This gap in interests seems to be reappearing in a new guise.

I take the point that an incompetent doctor may practise for years without doing anything so disastrous that she or he comes to the attention of Council, while a, generally speaking, good doctor may have one appalling lapse which brings down a serious professional misconduct charge upon him or her. I also know that in some cases where there was a proven charge of serious professional misconduct, a review of the entire history of the doctor's performance might have changed the committee's conclusion from admonishment to suspension or erasure. What worries me is that outcome seems to have disappeared from the discussion. I trust that when the details of these proposals come forward the relationship between 'performance' and 'outcome' will be clearly spelled out. The crucial test of the procedures proposed will be whether they are really likely to ensure continued competence.

Undoubtedly there is a major question of how performance is to be reviewed. But before that there is the question of preliminary screening, when it is decided whether a case should go forward for investigation. Merrison (1975, paragraphs 255–259) suggested that there should be a unit to investigate disciplinary cases to provide evidence for a prosecution, should one prove necessary. The committee approved the rather more active role in investigating complaints which the Council had adopted during Lord Cohen's presidency. As well as the more frequent meetings of the discipline committee which I have already noted, this included incurring

> considerable expense in collecting evidence and in prosecuting cases where it had received information which suggested that the conduct of a particular doctor should be investigated.
>
> *Merrison Report* (1975), paragraph 255

Not only did Merrison consider that this was a justified activity, the committee recommended an investigative unit rather than continuing the present practice of using private enquiry agents. A unit staffed by the GMC and under medical supervision would be able to get better information and in addition it would make the procedures more open, the committee felt. The Council successfully resisted this proposal and it was left out of the 1978 Act. The Merrison committee had clearly been right when it said

> We appreciate that the establishment of such a unit would be a matter of concern for the profession, whose members might well consider that a more active role by the GMC would be an unwelcome addition to the considerable amount of scrutiny to which their actions are already subject.
>
> *Merrison Report* (1975), paragraph 258

There is no discussion in the Merrison report of that other suggestion which is from time to time made, by Ian Kennedy (quoted in Smith, 1989b) and by Simanowitz (1990) on behalf of AVMA, namely that there should be an inspectorate which could routinely check on medical performance—whether or not a complaint had been made. Other professions and occupations are subject to independent inspection, after all. Such a proposal has always been implacably opposed by the medical profession; it goes right against the principle of professional self-regulation—and that had been defined as out with the Merrison committee's competence to discuss.

Kennedy has also suggested (Smith, 1989b) that the GMC should reregister doctors at regular intervals. This implies recertification by the licensing authorities. A former and greatly respected member of the Council told me he thought that was essential. At this time it seems to me doubtful whether the GMC proposals would include this, for I doubt if the profession would wear the trouble and expense involved. They are looking for other ways of checking continued competence. Where the knowledge base of a practice changes so often and so swiftly, recertification has much to commend it.

Clearly it will be necessary to scrutinize the proposals for competence and performance review when they finally emerge from the GMC very carefully to see just how well they seem likely to do the job which is needed. One of the questions which the GMC's working group has to consider in tightening the grip on competence is the relationship between complaints at the local level and the central GMC machinery. The proposals are to develop machinery modelled on the health committee machinery. In this case there would be panels of practitioners nominated by the Council in the various regions or districts throughout the country with responsibility to take preliminary action on behalf of the Council. Where a doctor's performance was in question they would presumably invite her or him to permit an examination of her or his practice over a period of time. In the case of the health committee, if a doctor is found, upon voluntary examination, to be unfit for practice by reason of ill health, mental or physical, she or he is requested to submit to supervised treatment and, if necessary, to cease to practice while she or he undergoes treatment. Only if the doctor either refuses to be examined or refuses to follow the necessary treatment regime is she or he referred to the health committee of the GMC, whereupon the formal procedures ensue.

What the parallel would be in incompetence cases is not quite clear. One can envisage that the panel members investigating the case might suggest that the doctor at once improved her or his practice in certain specified ways or that she or he entered into further education and training. In both cases she or he would be kept under review until the necessary improvements had been achieved. One can also envisage that refusal to co-operate would result in referral to a central 'performance' committee of the GMC. Questions of continued registration would undoubtedly arise. What is less clear is what the borderline might be between those cases which could be dealt with locally and those which were so serious they had to be referred forward at once. It is also not clear when and if incompetence or a severe adverse outcome would continue to be deemed a question of serious professional misconduct; indeed, whether at local and central level the Council would still deal only with potentially *serious* cases.

In health committee enquiries at the local level lay members are not at all involved. It is deemed to be a medical matter as to whether a doctor is sick or not and what treatment should be advised. A lay person is involved, however, on the health committee itself. There can be no question of it being a merely medical matter where alleged incompetence is concerned. Patients clearly have something here to say (but not everything that must be said) about the treatment they have received and its outcome. Lay persons undoubtedly have a part to play in performance reviews. How should the lay persons be chosen and to whom should they be accountable?

There is another difficult issue: this is the interface between this procedure, be it called incompetence or performance investigation, and the NHS procedures. What relationship will be proposed between the procedures relating to GPs or hospital doctors within the NHS and the new GMC procedure? This raises again the urgent need for a more co-ordinated system, a question to which I shall return later. From the patient point of view a single portal of entry, so that the complaint may be channelled from the outset in the most appropriate direction, would seem to be a minimum essential even before any further reforms are proposed.

The performance procedures will require legislation, whether by Orders in Council or amendment to the Medical Act 1983. As I argue below in the section where I discuss whether self-regulation can work, it would be regrettable if such changes were to be made without account being taken of the total array of regulatory procedures in health care.

Educational reform

Reference has already been made to the intention of the education committee to have another stab at the reform of the undergraduate curriculum. While the committee has authority over undergraduate medical education, its authority over other stages is less clear, as we have seen. How successful it may be this time round remains to be seen. That must depend not only on the committee's robustness and powers of persuasion, but also on how well convinced of the reforms needed other educational authorities now are. Sometimes external pressure can help.

Certainly there are serious challenges, in addition to the internal discontent within the profession itself about the state of medical education. Two of these exterior challenges were mentioned by the chairperson of the education committee in the *GMC Annual Report for 1989*. The first was the new secondary school curriculum, which is expected to mean that students reach medical school with even more enquiring minds than hitherto; the second the fall, for demographic reasons, in the number of available students over the next few years. A conference was called jointly by the Committee of Vice Chancellors and Principals (CVCP) and the GMC to discuss these problems. The conference was attended by medical school representatives and the main school teacher associations. On another front, clinical training will be affected by the reforms in the NHS. This requires continuing dialogue between the GMC and the NHS authorities to ensure continuing high standards of clinical training.

As we have seen (Chapter 9), although the committee has authority over basic medical education, it has not in the last decade been able to resolve the problems in the undergraduate curriculum, either as to its overcrowding or as to the mode of teaching. The education committee has failed in these tasks although it has long been acknowledged that cramming the medical student with facts is no longer relevant to either the modern world or modern medical knowledge and the rapid changes it undergoes. These problems are echoed in those of the pre-registration year. In part, as we saw, this has been because of a lack of co-ordination of all stages of medical education. The 1978 Act gave the education committee the responsibility to undertake that co-ordination, but no authority over any aspect beyond basic education. This weakness in the Act derived from the unwillingness of the royal colleges to cede any of their power. The president, in his *BMJ* response to Richard Smith's articles on the GMC, stressed the importance of consultation between the GMC and other bodies in educational innovation:

> I acknowledge here the great debt which it [the GMC] owes to the royal colleges as well as to the many other bodies involved, directly and indirectly, in undergraduate and postgraduate education and training.
>
> Kilpatrick (1989b), p. 111

But one suspects that, as things stand, the royal colleges may in effect have a power of veto.

Merrison had recommended that control of standards in specialist education should rest with the GMC through the specialist register which it should maintain. The GMC has put forward the possibility of a separate indicative specialist register, but what now seems to be coming about is the alternaitve, that is, the voluntary inclusion in the main register of specialist qualifications. Although presumably the GMC will have to be satisfied as to the standards of any qualification voluntarily registered, this arrangement will not give the Council the same authority over specialist qualifications which a statutory specialist register would provide. The GMC has none of the other powers which Merrison had thought necessary adequately to control specialist education, such as sending for the papers of accrediting bodies. Everything it does has to be based on voluntary co-operation and goodwill.

It would seem logical, if the GMC is to continue in roughly its present guise, that it should be given powers of control over all stages of medical education analogous to those which it has over basic medical education. Professor Rhodes, a Council member, has publicly suggested this (Rhodes, 1989).

A new Medical Act might be expected to contain such a provision. The GMC would, I think, be happier if it were better able to co-ordinate the whole of medical education, which would mean having more control of specialist education. Given the present mode of regulation the GMC has to try to take other bodies with it, including in the proposals for a new Medical Act. The fierce independence of the faculties and colleges is likely to continue. The moves which the GMC has taken in the last decade may be seen either as a softening-up process to prepare for greater changes to come or successful stalling by those, principally, I guess, the colleges and faculties, who do not want to lose power. Whether the variety of challenges which the education committee, the Council, and medicine more widely now face will lead to greater co-operation between the various educational bodies still remains to be seen. Past experience would suggest that just enough ground will be conceded to retain professional self-regulation, so that how much is yielded will depend on how heavy the pressure is felt to be.

Doctors qualified overseas

The Council's *1989 Annual Report* refers in two places to the working party established by the overseas committee to look into the possibility of establishing a single form of registration for overseas doctors, instead of differentiating between those whose primary qualifications come from overseas medical schools which are *recognized for full registration* and those which are *accepted for limited registration only*. The president also devoted a paragraph to this suggestion in his *BMJ* article, where he noted the change that the four-year restriction, regardless of registration status, imposed by government on the postgraduate study in the UK of overseas doctors, had made. The *Annual Report* gives no details about the working party or its lines of thinking. The minutes are not available at the time of writing.

There is a serious need for the Council to give a lead to show that it is entirely non-discriminatory in its registration procedures, as in all other matters. Until 1990 the overseas committee was still chaired by a white man. That year the committee was divided into three, the former subcommittees being given committee status. The overseas committee and committee F (which deals with full registration) are chaired by white men, but committee L, dealing with limited registration, is chaired in 1991 by Dr Admani, an overseas doctor. It is, of course as the president said when writing about a single form of registration for overseas doctors, 'obvious that we must not sacrifice quality of decision for speed of delivery' (*GMC Annual Report for 1989*, p. 2). This has to be true throughout the work of the Council. The Council still has a long way to go before one can be sure that it is giving the medical profession an appropriately anti-racist lead, so seriously needed in our troubled multi-racial society. It would be a totally new departure for the Council to do such a thing, but I believe it to be necessary in the name of good medicine.

More open government

I spoke earlier of the way in which regulators in a hierarchical system are necessarily removed from the reality of the lives of those they regulate as well as of those on whose behalf they undertake the regulation. Yet the legitimacy of the elite, its authority and power, depend upon the silences of those who do not participate, who are outside the process. Unless they accept what is being done it cannot be done. When the legitimacy is challenged, when the silences are broken, wise rulers meet their critics openly: I believe the GMC's troubles of 1968 and thereafter were compounded by secretiveness and defensive intransigence. The profession has no space in the 1990s to risk the disunity of a rift between medical leaders and front line practitioners, especially as open challenges to its legitimacy increase (I refer to appeals to the PC, and challenges in the courts and before tribunals).

This is not a conspiracy theory of medicine against the laity or of medical leaders against the rank and file of doctors. My belief has been that the regulation of the profession might work better, one hazard might be removed, if regulatory procedures were more open; if they involved a wider range of medical practitioners, a wider range of health workers and a wider range of persons who can represent patients and the public; and, finally, if there were much more and freer dialogue among all these categories on a basis of equality at every level of the service.

It seems that the GMC has learned part of this lesson. It has now established a press and publicity officer, where previously it gave the impression

of hiding from the press and feeling no need at all to communicate anything except the driest decisions. It has also in 1989 given a completely new
look to its *Annual Report*. Yet in the same year the president withdrew his
agreement to discuss the workings and policies of the GMC with Richard
Smith, who was writing a series of articles on the GMC for the *BMJ*. Sir
Robert insisted on writing an article himself (Lock, 1989). More careful
manipulation of the data available is not the same thing as making the
proceedings of Council clearly visible.

The president also says in the *GMC Annual Report for 1989* (p. 2) that the
Council has 'made determined efforts to forge links with organizations
representing patients' interests'. This is a great advance. One hopes that
the patients' organizations will be consulted on all aspects of the GMC's
work and not just on discipline. To invite representatives of lay bodies to
private lunch meetings with the president to discuss aspects of the GMC's
work is something earlier presidents did not do; formerly lay bodies were
not included in consultations. For patients' organizations there is the ever
present danger of co-option if meetings remain private. For any group
which has hitherto not been consulted and has for long been knocking on
the door to seek attention, such consultations are a great advance and no
doubt felt by some as flattering.

Furthermore, for real progress to be made, whether the meetings are
held in public, semi-public or privately, the Council (and other parties to
the discussions) have to move beyond the exchange of postures to genuine
exchanges of views and experiences on a basis of equality. Even in privileged meetings which I have attended I have not yet seen this happening.
It is in the long-term interests of the profession as well as the patients that
all the parties to health care provision should join together to solve
problems of mutual interest. I note that in the article quoted, the president
made no mention of the sorts of links that the GMC has with other
health care organizations, bodies representing the many other health
occupations, for example.

Will the reforms proposed be sufficient?

The Council will proceed on its proposed reforms of education, conduct
and performance through the process of consultation and consensus. Consultations will go more widely than they used to do and on conduct at least
will include patients' organizations. But my guess is that if Council continues to work on a model of medical consensus, change will be an even
longer time coming than is usual. There is a wide gap between the views
of 'progressive' and 'conservative' medical practitioners about necessary
changes in education and conduct control (and also vested interests). The
gap between medical 'conservatives' and some patients' organizations and

public representatives is even wider. It seems likely that the GMC will ultimately propose reforms upon which it can get a professional consensus, the 'progressives' perhaps using the patients' arguments to push the 'conservatives' further than they would otherwise go. The reforms are consequently unlikely to meet everyone's demands, but the question we have to ask here is whether they will go far enough to convince government and Parliament or far enough to ensure an adequately regulated profession.

Some form of regulation necessary

There is wide agreement that the medical profession does require regulation. Critics from right and left may suggest the abolition of the GMC and its replacement, for example, by a consumer-dominated body. No one, not even Green (1985), the right radical, has yet suggested that medicine can be entirely left to free market forces. The particular nature of the doctor–patient relationship, its intimacy and the associated potential for exploitation is one reason; the irremediable and serious nature of mistakes that can be made is another. 'Buyer beware' is little help to the irreparably damaged or dead person—the ultimate risk of falling into the wrong hands in the medical market. It is also clear that, unless all medicine were under the purview of the NHS, its regulation cannot rely on NHS procedures. Currently there is an increase in private practice; realistically there always will be private practice. Either, therefore, there would have to be two systems, one for those in private practice and one for those in state employ, or the primary regulation of the profession must be independent of the NHS. There are many reasons why it would be undesirable to have a dual system, not least because it might tend to two standards of practice. There are good ethical reasons for suggesting that there should be equality for all patients in the minimum standards of care they may expect from registered practitioners. Furthermore, in no other way could the unity of the profession be sustained.

What sort of body should be responsible for ensuring this minimum standard and how should it go about its work? In answering this question much must depend on what one thinks such a body should do. This in turn depends on how one thinks health care should be delivered, how much and what sort of part the state should play in that. Furthermore, proposals which only look upon the GMC as a complaints machinery are likely to take a different view from those which accept that a GMC should also control entry to the profession.

Rudolph Klein, writing in 1973, proposed a Council of the Professions— he accepted the professional mode. It was not then under any challenge and he wrote in that knowledge. He was concerned to improve the administrative checks on the way professional self-regulation worked. He was really looking at the GMC as part of the administrative complaints procedure and was concerned with efficiency in the delivery of health care as well as ensuring justice for patients. Klein believed that the best guarantee of an effective system of individual accountability is an effective system of collective accountability (Klein, 1973, p. 63).

His Council on the Professions would provide for interchange of information among the various councils of the self-regulating professions; could compare what each of the professions was doing in the way of evaluating the quality of services being delivered by its members and in ensuring their continued competence; and regular reviews would also show what professions were doing to develop the principle of public accountability (Klein, 1973, p. 163).

Klein is silent on how his Council should be composed or to whom *it* should be accountable. The Privy Council is probably the only office which at present has anything like an overview of the way professions and trades are regulated. It is also unclear what 'teeth' his Council might have as he himself implicitly acknowledges in a footnote (Klein, 1973, p. 64, fn. 18).

A more radical approach is the right-wing one of returning the professions to the market, thereby increasing consumer choice and breaking the professions' monopoly power. This preference for market control rather than state control or professional self-regulation clearly lay behind the government's green paper on restrictive practices. In Chapter 13 I discussed Green's proposals for removing the monopoly of the medical profession, controlling fraud in health care through the courts, and abolishing the GMC and replacing it with a body with more limited tasks, for he like other believers in the market still thinks medicine needs some regulation. The body would be non-medical and its members would have the legal status of trustees, liable in law for failure to discharge their duties correctly and forbidden to profit from their activities as trustees.

An earlier proposal for the abolition of the GMC came from the radical left in a memorandum submitted to the Merrison committee in the early 1970s by the Medical Practitioners Union (MPU). This recommended replacing the GMC by a body of consumers. The MPU's proposals assumed the continued existence of a publicly funded health care system available to all. Underlying notions were not of buyers and sellers of health care in an open market, or of producers and consumers, but rather of service providers and service users. Rather than thinking of themselves either as professionals entitled to special privileges, or as producers selling goods to consumers, the MPU of the early 1970s thought of medical practitioners as technicians, offering technical services and having no more power or rights than other technicians might have (Faulkner, personal communication). Within this context their proposals included one to ensure that practitioners should be protected from patients.

These proposals from radical right and radical left derive from diametrically opposed philosophies: the first is individualistic, where the second is collectivist; so the first argues for the delivery of health care in as free a market as possible, while the second thinks of health care as a social service provided as of right to the total population. The first denies the notion of collective responsibility and action while the second thinks in terms of the collective rights and duties of a particular occupation: their common denial of 'profession' is thus quite differently founded. The essential similarities between them are that both are opposed to the principle of professional self-regulation, both accept the specialness of medicine and its need for regulatory machinery, and both think this should be in lay control. Other than these two radical proposals, I have seen no worked-out proposals for the reform of the entire GMC functions and none from the left wing, although I understand that the MPU are working on the question in 1991. Any proposals will be unlikely, however, to follow the mid-1970s model.

A view from the patients' perspective

Distrust of self-regulation is not confined to the radical left and radical right. The Association of Community Health Councils of England and Wales (ASCHCEW), with experience of guarding the public interest so far as the health service is concerned, does not believe self-regulation provides appropriate safeguards. Dissatisfied with the present NHS complaints machinery, ASCHCEW (1988) proposed an independent complaints investigation service with medical advice but under lay control. ASCHCEW has offered a model of what it thinks an acceptable body to deal with patients' complaints in the NHS would be. This obviously does not constitute a blueprint for a revised GMC, even if one thought a reformed GMC should be the pinnacle of a complaints procedure—contrary to most present medical opinion, for ASCHCEW's model does not deal with issues of qualifications for practice or competence to continue in practice. However, it is an interesting indication of just how far, under the guidance of self-regulation, present procedures are from what patients' representatives find acceptable and what their concerns are.

ASCHCEW calls it a user's model which it offers for discussion. The model proposes:

1. clear information be available to the public regarding complaints, including what route to take for what sort of complaint;
2. time limits for the conclusion of any proceedings;

3. resources provided to support complainants;
4. an early investigation in each case to establish whether conciliation is an appropriate route or whether formal machinery should be invoked at once;
5. an 'independent complaints investigation service' with medical advice but under lay control to which complainants should have right of access;
6. all NHS medical practitioners to be under a contractual requirement to take part in grievance procedures;
7. complainants should receive a full explanation of the outcome of any enquiries;
8. a compensation agency to settle claims without prejudice to right of appeal to a Court if the compensation awarded were not satisfactory;
9. referral to professional bodies where necessary if professional disciplinary action seemed to be called for, the complainant being informed thereof;
10. the administrators of the new system should themselves be accountable.

The model assumes the continued existence of professional regulatory bodies, but as things stand such a proposal (quite apart from what might be government's view of its financial implications) is unlikely to be acceptable to the medical profession—if only because of its insistence on a lay body with medical advice, rather than medical determination.

But would it be so seriously against the profession's interests? Could it even be in the professional interest? Answers must depend on how one defines professions and professionalism.

Can self-regulation work?

Professional self-regulation may not be acceptable to the radical right or the radical left, but there is plenty of evidence that the principle is still acceptable to many people. Other occupations continue to follow the model of the GMC or wish they could do so. Social workers, discontented with what they see as the partiality of local authority enquiries, are one such contemporary group.

Smith recognized that there was an underlying question as to whether the self-regulation of doctors is still acceptable (Smith, 1989b). However, a crucial question is whether his criticisms of the GMC are not *really criticisms of professional self-regulation itself*? Certainly David Bolt *et al.* saw that danger, for the bulk of their letter contained the following *credo*:

> Above all we wish to affirm that there is a very substantial majority view among members of the BMA favouring the central principle of professional

self regulation, while fully supporting the essential safeguard that such regulation must, in a free society, be undertaken with the benefit of lay opinion
and advice such as that which the lay members of the Council provide. We
also venture to suggest that this principle would, if seriously challenged, be
firmly endorsed by an informed body of public opinion.

                                                        Bolt et al (1989), p. 1125

Unreasoned and unsupported arguments of this kind had kept the principle off the agenda of the Merrison committee. Sir Robert Kilpatrick
(Kilpatrick, 1989c) put a more reasoned case, including the important point
that 'self imposed discipline is much more likely to be accepted by
members of the profession than that imposed from outside'. This, however, overlooks the question of just how far 'outside' their everyday lives
many members of the profession practising in Britain feel the GMC to be,
remote as it still appears, unrepresentative of women, young doctors, non-
white doctors as it is. Sir Robert further says that he is sure that no doctor
who understands what the principle is all about would wish to lose it and
continues 'the GMC will continue to *assert* and uphold the principle' (my
emphasis). If the failures of the GMC which Smith pointed to are failures
of self-regulation itself then the GMC will not be capable of rising to the
challenges which are now facing it.

Stephen Lock (Lock, 1989), in an editorial which followed Richard
Smith's articles, called for another enquiry into the role of the GMC 'in
both regulation and education', saying, with a bit of exaggeration, that it
was almost 20 years since the subject was examined in depth. Lock suggests the profession itself should set up the enquiry, because of the importance of self-regulation, but that it would be better if it was an independent
rather than an internal inquiry. He concludes his editorial by pointing out
that a GMC which fulfilled its functions properly would be a good deal
more expensive, but that doctors should be prepared to pay

> both because the benefits will be correspondingly greater (to doctors and to
> society) and because they need to keep regulation of the profession where it
> belongs—with the profession.

That call was made in July 1989. There is no indication that the GMC have
any intention of proposing an independent enquiry.

My analysis suggests that professionalism as developed in the medical
profession may make it impossible to achieve appropriate regulation by the
profession. Both the need to maintain unity, in order to self-regulate and
the loyalty to the concept of the greater profession, over and above sectional medical interests called forth to sustain that unity tend to restrict and
retard what the GMC can do. The felt need to consult and consult again

in order to reach consensus decisions greatly slows down the decision-making process. Indeed the procedures may either transform the proposals away from their original intention or hold them up indefinitely, an effective veto. The institutionalization of control in a series of elite groups which have many of their own internal problems to deal with, reduces the sensitivity of their members to what it happening 'out there' and their ability to understand what they hear.

The great advantage of professional self-regulation, when those doing the regulating are sufficiently in touch with the general body of the professionals, is the greater acceptability of self-imposed regulation. Even given the inevitable gap between leaders and led, there it something different about having 'one of us' giving out orders rather than a 'rank outsider' who 'just doesn't understand'. Membership of a self-regulating profession is likely to increase the sense of worth of it members and, given appropriate working conditions, this is likely to enhance the standard of their work. The service ethic, an essential part of medical professionalism, is another major inherent (if sometimes rather latent) advantage.

Professional self-regulation, as we have seen, permeates all aspects of medical regulation, including the law, where medical evidence, unlike evidence from all other professions and occupations, is determinative, not advisory. There is a sense in which the GMC is the standard bearer for medical professionalism, and for that it takes a lot of stick. However, it cannot, as an institution, be held responsible for all the wide array of medical accountability procedures and practices.

The GMC can suggest reforms of its own procedures and practices and request legislation to that end; it may, through committees on which its president or other representative sits, propose changes in, for example, the NHS disciplinary or complaints procedures (as it did in relation to the proposed new NHS discipline procedures); but it is not responsible for the NHS, nor for the operation of the law. Nevertheless, what the GMC does sets the tone for the profession. The reforms it initiates may well have repercussions in other parts of the system. Furthermore, its own responsibilities for regulating the profession give it some authority to make statements about how other facets of the regulatory process help or hinder its own task.

There is professional as well as lay discontent with many aspects of medical accountability, not least with medical negligence. John Havard, the secretary of the BMA, in the 1989 Stephens Lecture to the laity at the Royal Society of Medicine, reviewed the associated problems: the burden of proof, the adversarial system of justice, various proposals for reform contingency, no-fault compensation and other remedies and solutions to this 'mounting dilemma'. He concluded by saying that he thought a comprehensive review was needed

> by a body with powers to requisition information about settlements which
> cannot be made public, and with the capability of taking into account all the
> interests involved, not least the constitutional rights of the citizen, which
> must be balanced against the need to protect our health service from damage.
>
> Harvard (1989a), p. 27

Not only is there discontent with all the individual components of the accountability procedure but the system as a whole is held by many to be working badly. It is not really a *system* of accountability: it is an array which, like Topsy, 'just growed'. The trouble is not simply that the GMC as at present constituted is not able fully to ensure the competence of registered practitioners, although this is the case; or that the law does not work well for any of the parties involved; or that the NHS disciplinary machinery creaks. The many components which comprise the total regulatory system are badly co-ordinated, leading to confusion for both practitioner and patient. The system is in need of reform and rationalization, as the discussion in Chapter 14 (pp. 215–216) showed.

Since John Havard gave the Stephens lecture there have been further moves in the direction of establishing no-fault compensation. Crown indemnity has been introduced, so that NHS doctors are no longer personally responsible for claims through their own medical insurance. There has been a working party on reform of the NHS medical staff disciplinary procedures. The GMC is working towards reform of *its* disciplinary procedure. Each of these things has been done without (so far as is publicly known) any reference to how it might relate to other aspects of medical accountability. Topsy is 'just grow'd-ing' even further. The upshot will be a change in the nature of medical regulation without the principle on which it is based ever having really been examined.

An enquiry needed

The time has come to look at the entire UK system of regulation of the medical profession as a whole rather than reviewing and reforming its component parts in a piecemeal manner. An independent enquiry should look not only at the GMC, as Lock suggested, or at medical negligence issues, as Havard suggested, but the wider issues of the regulation and accountability of the profession and all the institutions involved. Such an enquiry would look at the component parts, how they are articulated together, including where the GMC fits into that. But above all the enquiry should look at professional self-regulation to establish the balance of advantages and disadvantages it offers. Why has the profession always been so shy, since they are convinced it is so manifestly a good principle, of having self-regulation examined? Dare one whisper that that might be because they know it really is better for the profession than for the public, that its principal purpose is to maintain their power and status?

Given the close-knit interdependence of all health care occupations, it may be that the enquiry should look at regulation and accountability right across the health care professions. Certainly it is unreal that discipline, where blunders may have been made by members of more than one profession, e.g. nurses and technicians as well as doctors, should be looked at in isolation by each profession in turn as is now the case. The case for dealing with each profession separately depends on the very principle of self-regulation which it would be the first task of the enquiry to examine. This suggests the enquiry should proceed by stages, first examining professional self-regulation. If this should fail, then the subsequent proceedings would follow the course of looking at the regulation of health care professions as a whole. If it were upheld, separate enquiries as to professional regulation for each health care occupation would then be in order.

What kind of regulatory body is needed?

Such an enquiry would need to start by considering what kind of regulatory body is needed. My studies have led me to conclude that an adequate system of regulation should take account of the interests of the practitioners, those they work with and their patients. The criteria by which one might judge whether any medical profession is really well-regulated may be said to include the following:

1. that the profession ensures that only appropriately qualified doctors are admitted to practice;
2. that those continuing in practice are competent;
3. that they work conscientiously;
4. that those allowed to practise do not exploit their patients economically, socially or sexually;
5. that those allowed to practise do not exploit their colleagues or subordinates;
6. that patients or their representatives have ready access to the regulatory body in case of the alleged failure of a practitioner in any of these respects;
7. that patients or their representatives should receive equitable and adequate compensation for any damage resulting from medical accident or misdemeanour;
8. that practitioners are afforded appropriate protection against wrongful actions of patients, employers, colleagues or others.

Would those characteristics be agreed as important by professionals and patients at large? All practitioners would agree that those in practice should be appropriately qualified, competent and work conscientiously; also that they should not exploit patients in any way. Practitioners would agree with not exploiting colleagues at least in the sense of not disparaging them. Little attention has been paid in professional codes to the exploitation of subordinates. Ready access by patients to regulatory bodies is not something which in the past the profession has been too pleased to offer. It is almost as if, as Smith implies (Smith, 1989f, p. 1502; i, p. 42), patients and the public are seen as the enemy; however, I imagine that in principle this criterion would be conceded. So far as individual cases are concerned one can expect dispute and challenge about damage and compensation, but a professional body, at least theoretically, could surely only be in agreement as to the justice of that criterion. It is unlikely that most patients would recognize that practitioners may need protection against them, but practitioners certainly will.

In thinking about these criteria it is clear that one must distinguish between individual professionals and the profession as a collectivity. This distinction has constantly cropped up in the preceding discussions. It is clearly in the interests of the profession as a collectivity to provide as good a service as modern knowledge, skill and technology can offer; to achieve that may be difficult for any one individual practitioner, for a whole host of reasons. In principle the interests of patients and the profession do not diverge; in practice they often do—from a patient's need for a house call in the early hours of the morning to much more serious issues. Herein lies one of the problems of self-regulation in practice as opposed to in principle.

Does all or part of the regulatory system fulfil these criteria at present? Because the GMC is responsible for ensuring that members of the public can trust any registered medical practitioner whom they consult—which it does by maintaining a register of those fit to practise—it is also responsible for criteria: (1) appropriate qualifications, (2) competence of those in practice, (3) their conscientiousnes and (4) no exploitation of patients. The third could be argued to be a matter of wise patient choice, but, given the specialness of medicine, could also reasonably be said to be part of proper professional practice. Given that the GMC has to maintain the register of the competent it could also be said by implication to be responsible for (6), ready access; otherwise, how may it know that its register is reliable? Characteristic (7), compensation, is right outside the GMC's present tasks—it falls to the law. The GMC deals with a small part of (8), protection of practitioners, namely where damage to medical colleagues offends the ethical guidelines, but for the most part the medical trade unions and defence societies and sometimes the law are responsible.

In practice the GMC does not fulfil these tasks at all adequately at present, as we have seen. In addition a number of other authorities—the NHS, other employing authorities—are involved in all except (1), i.e. ensuring that only appropriately qualified doctors are permitted to practise. The GMC has, furthermore, rested very heavily on the NHS procedures, something for which Jean Robinson has criticized it roundly. The NHS procedure are, of course, no help to patients in private practice who have only the GMC or the law to turn to. Aggrieved patients do not have ready access to the GMC (criterion 6).

A main problem is that professions, including the medical profession, do not think in terms of the kind of regulatory body which I have outlined above. The nature of professionalism as presently understood stands on different premises and ones which I argue are not in the best interests of the profession or its clients. For these reasons, in the next chapter I argue that a new kind of professionalism is needed.

17

Towards a
New Professionalism

A new kind of professionalism

Historically sociologists have been divided between those who see the professions as of great advantage to the development of a good society and the maintenance of social stability and those who have stressed the considerable power of the professions and point to ways in which that power has been misused. The latter view has tended to dominate over the last two decades. Many of the sociological arguments about the power of the professions might seem to support the notion that the medical profession as a highly privileged self-regulating body should be dismantled.

Either way, old-style professionalism has had its day. The conditions in which it was created have changed out of all recognition. Modern health care is now a complex and major industrial enterprise; it is no longer a cottage industry. The patient no longer has a relationship with one doctor, but with one (and possibly more) backed by many support staff, and perhaps also including other independent professionals such as clinical psychologists or social workers. A more highly educated populace demands more information and requests more involvement in the treatment.

The tight professional organization, its exclusiveness, its seeming arrogance have engendered too much hostility for medicine to be able to continue as it is. The strong market domination of health care, which its professional organization has helped it to achieve, attracts criticism from many more than the radical right with their belief in the value in all circumstances of free market forces. It attracts opposition from practitioners of other healing modes as well as from those occupations which medicine has subordinated in the division of health labour. Increasingly patients are unprepared to accept the subservient position medicine has historically accorded them.

If medicine attempts to hang on to the old model of professionalism and to preserve as many of the sacred cows as possible, I fear that, not only may professional self-regulation be swept away, but also that the best of professionalism, its valuable aspects, will be lost along with those parts which need to go. The end result could be different from anything anybody intended and have unwanted consequences for the profession and public. Better that the profession itself should recognize the need for radical change; that medical leaders themselves should establish a new concept of profession within which the best of the old model could be preserved, while modifying the concept to fit the new circumstances.

The public value of a strong medical profession

There are, furthermore, certain cogent arguments against the proposal that medicine as a powerful profession should be dismantled (Stacey, 1988b). They fall under two headings, those relating to the good of the public end those relating to the good of the profession, although each feeds into the other. A major advantage from the public point of view of a strong and united profession is that it can oppose government proposals or actions when necessary in the interests of the health of the people. Would a de-regulated profession be likely, or able successfully, to do that? The already fragile unity of what is now a very diverse and highly differentiated profession might well not survive de-regulation. Given the addition of an NHS based on principles of competition rather than co-operation and service, the interests of different individuals and occupational segments within medicine could well become paramount. This presents the prospect that the strong and independent body, able to speak for the public health, would be lost.

The theory and practice of medicine has had many beneficial consequences. The power of the professions, while generally exercised in a most conservative and self-interested manner, has, from time to time, been pitted against reactionary proposals, for example proposals to make abortion law more restrictive or in defence of the NHS. Scientific pronouncements of epidemiologists have drawn attention to deficiencies in the government's public health policies, e.g. with regard to salmonella, listeriosis, nuclear power and waste. One can argue that it is in the interests of a centralizing government to weaken the organized profession as much as is consistent with retaining the services of the professionals themselves, for the government has need of a healthy nation.

Centralization as well as free market

While the Thatcher government's arguments for clipping professional wings are couched in terms of the free market, it would be naive to consider deregulation proposals simply in those terms. Rather, deregulation has to be seen in the context of a government which, while professing liberal values of free competition and private enterprise, has strengthened central government control in many aspects of life in a manner unprecedented in Britain: controls which interfere with free speech, the media, education and research.

In the course of this centralizing process, all those structures with political power and resources sufficient to oppose or obstruct government programmes have been systematically tamed and weakened. Structures which came between the individual citizen and the state, such as trade unions, local government, the universities, have all been diminished and restrained in this way. Seen in this context the government's programme to curtail the power and privileges of the profession emerges in rather a different light.

Fortunately, total deregulation seems unlikely in practice, whatever the ideology of the government. Not only would it in some ways work against the public interest as noted above, but from the professional point of view the occupation would then also rapidly lose a coherent vision of its *own* collective good. Rather than total deregulation, a reduction in professional autonomy is more likely—indeed this is already beginning to happen to some extent in the reorganized NHS.

Professional self-reform

These arguments suggest that in the interests of medicine itself, as well as of the public that it serves, the profession needs to take a good deal further the self-reforms which it has already initiated in a number of areas, in education, competence, audit, for example. The facet of professionalism in medicine which works well towards good regulation is the service ethic. It is to this that I think both profession and public must look for the future. From this a new professionalism may be developed which will be appropriate for the twenty-first century.

Just as a main advantage of self-regulation is that regulation from peers is likely to be more acceptable than regulation from outside, so there are major advantages for the profession in undertaking its own reform. Medicine as an occupation was a prime leader in establishing the concepts of profession and professionalism. It is now in a good position to lead the way towards the new professionalism which other service occupations could follow.

The new professionalism would realize that the restrictive practices essential to establish the profession in the nineteenth century are now no longer needed. Medicine is well entrenched as the leading healing mode, although to practitioners and professional leaders, who receive the flak that flies against their practice and profession, may not feel so secure. Medicine is, however, much stronger than its collective paranoia permits it to see.

In thinking about this new professionalism two aspects have to be borne in mind: the individual, practitioner–patient aspect and the collectivity of the profession as a whole. Work has to be done on both counts. Already at the practitioner level a great deal of work has gone on which is laying the foundations for this new professionalism. Medical knowledge, for example, is shared with patients and the public much more freely than it used to be. Many GPs work with or refer their patients to complementary or alternative healers, such as acupuncturists. There are practices where the collegial relationships have been extended to include staff of all kinds. Some hospitals include many non-biomedical healers and counsellors among the services they offer. Numbers of doctors are seeking to establish relationships of greater equality with their patients.

However, the dominant professional ethos, the kind of training many young doctors still receive and the rules and guidance that are offered to practitioners, too frequently still act as a deterrent to such developments. In any case, it is not enough just to change some relationships in this way, although that is important. The collective ethos also has to change so that good developments are no longer shackled.

Tasks towards the new professionalism

The first task in working towards the new professionalism is to ensure that the profession puts the patient and the collectivity of patients not necessarily *first*, but equal to and part of the professional interest. The patients can be, and historically have been, the profession's greatest ally, not only providing work (patients are, after all, the *sine qua non* of the profession) but often providing support in time of trouble. The loyalty that I have seen patients express in the GMC when pleading for their own doctors— including some really rascally ones—to be permitted to continue to practise should reassure practitioners. Those who have had cause for complaint and some other members of the public may be less happy.

To serve the patient well, to put the patient above personal and sectional interests, is already the ideal. In practice, under the old professionalism it has not really worked out that way, as I have shown. In its own interest the profession would be wise to work through all necessary facets to check that it really is providing a good service, both as a collectivity in what it aims to do and so far as the performance standards of its members are concerned. To achieve this the profession will have to listen to what patients say and to understand the way they see things—their conceptual framework.

Medical exclusiveness, one of the now unnecessary restrictive practices, has also to yield in relation to other health care professions. The equality of importance of all other health care workers has to be recognized, their different but essential input. In addition to joining with such professionals to regulate the health care enterprise, uncomfortable questions will also have to be asked about differentials in status and remuneration. Although even top-rank British doctors are less affluent than colleagues in the USA and parts of Europe, differentials between them and other health workers have been too large for too long.

How quickly can the new professionalism develop?

As professional leaders have already recognized, there is not much time to waste. It will take time, however, to change old ideas, especially ones, such as clinical autonomy and self–regulation, so firmly embedded during initial training and by subsequent repetition. The first step must be to move towards what the profession thinks it already has been doing—seeing that all registered practitioners are reasonably competent. This goal is beginning by some to be seen as more important than blind and unthinking collegial loyalty—as expressed in the ethical guidelines. The importance, for example, of medical audit is recognized by all practitioners who want to see a good job done and who are motivated by the service ethic. Many are not yet convinced and, no doubt, the conviction expressed by some may be mere lip service.

It is understandable that medical practitioners should wish to draw a clear distinction between audit for financial reasons and audit to ensure high standards of practice. It is also understandable that at this stage the profession, only segments of which have hitherto undertaken any systematic reviews of their practice, should insist on audit being closed to any one other than fellow professionals. Those professions which medicine has subordinated understandably wish to undertake their own reviews without medical interference. I would hope, however, that as the new professionalism develops audits would be opened up, not only to other health care workers (for, as I keep saying, so much health care is a joint enterprise with shared responsibility), but also to patients who, after all, in most cases make an active input to their own treatment.

Time must be allowed for the changes at all levels to take place. However, what the profession urgently needs to do is to show that the changes it is proposing are not merely defensive—to change as little as possible and to retain as much power as possible—but that it recognizes that a new kind of professionalism is now needed. If the profession is unable to make such an earnest of intention and to articulate a schedule of the goals to be achieved and how quickly movement can follow, then others are likely to develop the goals and the schedule for the profession. If the profession does not itself set up such a programme it will be because diehards in places of power will not permit it. And here we are back to the problems of self–regulation. However, the GMC, with its statutory responsibilities, its unique understanding of the profession as a whole, is in a position to give such a lead.

Changes needed to create the new professionalism

What the new professionalism will mean is that the profession will have to respond in free and open discussion to the demands of other groups, that proposals will be made and modified, new boundaries drawn and negotiations continued. In some ways this is, of course, what already happens—except for the 'free and open' bit. Negotiations now take place among elites, sometimes reported, sometimes not. Patients' groups are now being included in these negotiations much more than ever before. This is a great advance, but those groups, and particularly their leaders, will have to take care they themselves are not co-opted to the elite system.

Education for the new professionalism

What about the type of education which practitioners should receive? To make way for the new professionalism artificial and inhibiting divisions in medicine will have to be superseded by a more genuine collegiality. Factions within medicine seem to have been deadlocked for too long on the relationship of the various stages of education to each other. The mode of education of young doctors in hospital, modelled essentially on the old professionalism, has been a major factor in undermining that very concept of professionalism. Once junior hospital doctors were granted overtime pay, the old concept of profession received a major dent from within the profession itself.

The damage arose from internal contradictions within medicine whereby the equality of all fully qualified practitioners, strongly upheld, contrasted with the subordinate role of all those in training grades. The carrot, that they would one day achieve full professional status, was not enough for junior hospital doctors in the often alienating conditions of the modern hospital. They took the trade union rather than the professional route to solve their problems. The discomforts of their position again, at the end of 1990, threatened the unity of the profession and the running of the hospital service itself, leading to government intervention (see Chapter 9, pp. 122–123).

The old professionalism failed to solve this problem. A new professionalism would recognize and totally review the conditions of training of young doctors and their relationship to their chiefs as well as to the NHS;

indeed, the concept of 'chiefs' itself may well need review. It has to be recognized that the grievances of the junior hospital doctors, while they are exacerbated by the problems facing the NHS as a result of under-funding and reorganization, are in essence created by an old professionalism, deeply imbued with ideas of status and essentially traditonal in outlook ('what was good enough for my father ...'; 'I went through it, so can they...'). More appropriate training conditions would improve service to the patients and reduce the disadvantages which young doctors with responsibility for young children incur. The current conditions of work were devised for an all-male profession where the men undertook no domestic responsibilities. Special conditions for women are not what is needed, but civilized working hours and a less punitive rota or shift system for all junior hospital doctors.

One of the crucial times and places where the values of the old professionalism are instilled into the young practitioner is during the training by chiefs in hospital. A new set of relationships and structures would go along with teaching the more open values of the new professionalism.

Lay involvement in educational control?

Should the control of medical education continue to remain entirely in professional hands? Only the trained have the skills to judge the technical competence of entrants to the profession, but there are other facets where the non-medically qualified have a contribution to make. Educational experts can contribute on topics such as selection of students, examination procedures and teaching methods. Patients and potential patients can comment on the broad outlines of the education medical students receive. For example, a medical training was not needed to observe that, until very recently, doctors were trained in and given experience almost exclusively of hospital medicine while patients most often consulted GPs. That has now been remedied by including general practice as a specialty in the clinical training and the pre-registration year and also by requiring by law vocational training for all intending GPs. Lay advice would have put those advances sooner rather than later: they do not need to be told that most consultations are with GPs and that the quality of their practitioner is of the essence. One cannot always wait for professionalizing ambitions (in this case those of GPs which led to these changes) to catch up with problems patients experience.

So far as the deadlock about putting together all stages of medical education is concerned, it is possible that, had there been a stronger voice from other health care workers and from patients and potential patients, the deadlock might already have been broken. Patients and potential patients have a strong interest in these issues, for the quality of medical care is undoubtedly affected by them and most patients receive a great deal of their treatment from doctors in various stages of training. The problems of junior hospital doctors crucially affect other health care workers also, particularly nurses.

Control of entry to the profession has been one of the cornerstones of the old concept of professionalism. Where would it fit into the new? Again, following from the criteria of what a well-regulated profession would look like, the already qualified practitioners and the educators would clearly have a major input to make as to what is a properly qualified practitioner. Theirs is the technical knowledge and the practical experience. But, as in the content of the education deemed necessary and the conditions of training, there is a legitimate view from other health care professionals and from patients and potential patients.

How would the new professionalism regulate medicine?

A revised composition for the GMC

A first step would be to propose some crucial changes in the structure and powers of the GMC. Measures to ensure adequate representation of young doctors, women and ethnic minorities would be urgently needed—not simply so that the GMC might appear more representative, but also so that the contribution of all those categories of doctors to the health of the nation, whether in private practice or the NHS, should be fully, fairly and equally taken into account in the Council's deliberations.

The new professionalism would recognize the status of other qualified health care professionals and would accord them adequate places on the Council as of right. The unique contribution they can make by reason of their training and practice experience to the regulation of the profession, both its educational and its disciplinary aspects, would thereby be recognized.

The new professionalism would also wish to seek greatly to increase the proportion of non-medical members on the Council. It would drop the term 'lay', which comes from the out-dated idea of exclusive and esoteric, not to say mystical, knowledge. In their wisdom the new professionals would probably finally decide that all the non-medically qualified taken together should constitute rather more than half of the membership in order to ensure that the service ethic remained to the fore.

A vigorous lead

A new GMC, so constituted, would continue to consult with other medical bodies, as it now does, but would be more vigorous in giving a lead to the profession. It would also restrict more tightly the time and number of these rounds of consultation and would not be afraid to make proposals which might run against the interests of some. It would be more vigorous in its inspection of educational bodies. Legislation would be needed to do these things and, in seeking that, the self-reforming GMC would request stronger powers over all stages of medical education and would propose a specialist register, rather than the voluntary inclusion of special qualifications in the present register.

One body or more?

Thought would have to be given as to whether the functions which the GMC now performs and the enhanced functions I have suggested it should undertake can reasonably be performed by one body. Controlling educational standards and entry qualifications is a large and demanding task and one which is distinct from ensuring that those on the register remain competent to practise. The two functions could be said to overlap at the point of the uptake of continuing medical education. However, to ensure the provisions are there, to indicate what continuing education should be received, when and by whom, is an educational function; to see that practitioners comply with the conditions laid down is a different and disciplinary function. There is no logical reason why the register should not be retained by one authority, the educational standard be set by another and the disciplinary functions as to fitness to practise in relation to continuing competence, appropriate general behaviour and health be carried out by a third.

A matter for discussion

This is not the place to draw up a blueprint for what the profession might wish to do in the course of reforming itself, or to offer detailed advice to all those non-medical bodies who would undoubtedly wish to make an input into the discussion. Rather I shall just outline some of the issues that will have to be considered. In thinking about these it will also be important to remember to work out how the many facets of medical regulation interface with each other.

Legal or administrative justice?

There have in the past been suggestions that the functions performed by the GMC should be divided. Many have seen it as inappropriate that the Council should be prosecutor, judge and jury in disciplinary cases. Marilyn Rosenthal (1987) has suggested the Swedish model whereby representatives of all health care occupations sit with non-health-qualified representatives to judge cases of alleged misconduct. By implication she is suggesting that discipline should be dealt with separately.

The complexity and interdependence of all facets of modern medicine lend force to arguments which suggest that all health care occupations should be controlled by one overarching regulatory body. Sweden has a much smaller population than the UK. An overarching body which dealt with all the regulatory facets of the present GMC would be likely to lead to a top-heavy bureaucracy simply because of size. In this case to separate discipline from other functions would make good sense. One body responsible for professional conduct, fitness and competence issues across the health care professions has much to commend it. However, the volume of work in the UK would be likely to require revolution to regions, even so.

The Rosenthal proposal is for a system of administrative justice to handle what she, in United States parlance, refers to as 'medical malpractice'. Others have proposed that lawyers should take over the disciplinary functions of the GMC, judging cases where the GMC alleged serious professional misconduct (or whatever charge might later supersede that). While this would avoid the accusations of 'prosecutor, judge and jury' to which the GMC is at present open, it would not necessarily meet some of the problems which I have raised in this book. The adversarial system whereby cases are tried in the GMC does not produce the best possible results and would not necessarily be made any better by having a lawyer in a controlling rather than an advisory position as at present. Other legal models, increasingly being thought about in the UK, which avoid the adversarial mode could be used.

However, there is also the problem that the law is as remote from the daily lives of ordinary people as is medicine—and remote from medicine also. While lawyers are trained to make impartial judgements, the law, even with recent reforms, remains an old-style profession. Furthermore, there is also the problem that professionals tend to see things more from the rarified view of any elite rather than from the perspective of the everyday lives of most members of the public. Complete impartiality is hard to achieve. Finally, the law is expensive.

My own inclination would be for some form of administrative machinery controlled and operated by a body reformed along the lines on which I suggested above that the GMC should be restructured, i.e. to include non-medical health personnel and representatives of the patients and potential patients as well as representatives of the medical profession. But I would not want to be rigid about this. The important thing is that new machinery should be worked out in the spirit of the new professionalism and should take account of the basic principles of proper regulation which I outlined at the conclusion of the last chapter.

It would also be vital to work out how this machinery would fit with the NHS disciplinary and complaints procedures. At present there are so many ways that a doctor may be disciplined. Any one of them may bring her or him to the GMC on a charge of serious professional misconduct. The more this relationship can be streamlined and the findings of one body accepted without what amounts to a retrial, the better. This would get over the double jeopardy problems, so worrisome to all practitioners. The part to be played by the register is crucial here.

Education

Whether the body controlling education was part of the new GMC or not, it would not be consistent with the new professionalism that control should be almost entirely in the hands of the royal colleges and the universities as it is at present. The new professionals would see the importance of strong representation on the controlling body, not only of practising doctors but also of students, young doctors and the public (drawn from a wide range).

The register

The control of the register is the key to the control of the profession. The crucial points about it are that persons admitted in the first instance should be properly qualified; that any persons who have shown themselves to be demonstrably unfit to practise for whatever reasons should be removed; that the continuing competence of those remaining on the register is assured. This suggests the need for relicensure and for an inspectorate. It is not for me to suggest how these should be worked out, but it would be wise of the profession, in consultation with others, if they began to work on possible procedures.

Other parts of the regulatory system

These considerations show just how important it is that there should be free-flowing information between any regulatory bodies relating specifically to the profession and other regulatory bodies within the health care system. Again it is not my brief to prepare a blueprint for this but perhaps to indicate places where attention will need to be paid. The new professionalism would have certain immediate consequences in so far as the narrow interpretation of clinical autonomy would no longer apply.

The health service commissioner

One obvious example is the health service commissioner (HSC), who has responsibility for looking at complaints of maladministration in the NHS. The old professionalism has hobbled the commissioner's work because she or he is not allowed to look at matters which are protected by the doctrine of clinical autonomy. Commissioners have varied in how near to questions involving medical judgement they have been prepared to go, how far they have been prepared to ask, for example, whether a practitioner had put herself or himself in a position to make a sound judgement. Removal of that disability would sharpen up the NHS complaints procedure a great deal.

NHS complaints procedures

Careful arrangements would have to be made to relate the existing procedures for complaints which have a clinical component to the enlarged work of the HSC. Appeal to the HSC from those procedures for parties who felt that their difficulties had not been resolved is one possible route. The procedures themselves need review and strengthening in ways which the new professionalism would be prepared to permit. Their improvement, as well as increasing the HSC's role and reforming the profession itself, is important to restrain the rising levels of litigation. Many people do not want to sue for compensation: they just want an admission that something went wrong, an apology and an assurance that every effort will be made to prevent a repetition. However, there are those circumstances in which a person needs compensation, for example for a lost ability to earn or a lost breadwinner.

Compensation for medical damage

As we saw earlier, the current legal procedures are not a good way of adjudicating cases where patients or their relatives are seeking compensation for medical damage they allege they have received. There is increasing support for no-fault compensation: a bill, albeit without government support is on the parliamentary agenda. The disadvantage of this is that there is no assurance that the cause of the injury or accident will be sought out and removed, whether it lies in procedures, equipment or personnel.

To my mind a far better way of dealing with this problem would be to take up the proposal made by Ham *et al.* (1988) of providing compensation through social security. In this proposal the authors suggest that all accidents, of whatsoever kind, including medical accidents, should be compensated for as of right through the social security system. Compensation would be set by the extent and consequences for the victim of the injury received and not, as now, in the adversarial system of British law. The Ham *et al.* proposals have the merit of universality and equality—all victims would be automatically covered and in the same way—and, finally, if the provisions were properly administered, all would be assured ease of access.

How far, how fast?

Rapid progress to the new professionalism cannot be expected. Changes are likely to come about in a piecemeal fashion. The grand logical new design is not the British way. The continual and radical NHS reforms have not encouraged either practitioners or public to be happy with such wholesale approaches. Progressive elements in the profession—about 20% are committed to some progressive cause (Watkins, 1987)—will be pushing for change in the direction I have called 'the new professionalism'. The GMC has already set its face towards important changes in the area of competence—or performance as they prefer to call it.

Step One: an independent enquiry

Without a sudden conversion to the new professionalism, the existing GMC is before too long likely to call for a Medical Act to encompass the reforms it will wish to see; these may include stronger powers to control all stages of medical education, some better ways of handling competence and possibly the establishment of a separate specialist register. In my view government would be unwise to accede to such a request without there first having been an independent, preferably state-sponsored, enquiry into all aspects of the regulation of the medical profession and of medical accountability. It is to be hoped that government would find time for such a radical review and the subsequent necessary legislation. Piecemeal approaches to the question are one reason for the present unsatisfactory state of affairs.

I have said the profession would itself be wise to call for such an enquiry forthwith and one which would crucially examine the concept of professional self-regulation. The enquiry would weigh the advantages and disadvantages of that concept and the way it works and recommend what principles should in future guide the regulation of the profession.

In the public interest, as well as in its own interest, medicine needs to remain strong and united. Nothing I have said about the disadvantages of professional self-regulation should be taken as suggesting anything other. Any group of workers—and here medicine is no exception—is right to keep as much control over the working lives of its members as it can. By the same token no group of workers is entitled to do that at the expense of other workers, customers or clients.

Consequently I am looking to the profession for a vigorous lead towards a better mode of regulation. The GMC is uniquely placed to give such a lead by using its powers to the full, transforming itself and thus helping in the movement to the new professionalism which is so urgently needed.

Endnote

The service ethic can survive and flourish much better in some circumstances than in others. A fully expressed service ethic means that doctors (and all other health care workers) are able to make their services available to all who need them; that they do not have to think where the money is coming from either for the patient to pay or them to live on; that they can treat the condition whoever the patient may be. The service ethic was able to flourish well under the NHS as originally conceived where services were freely available to all as they were needed. Where competition and profit enter, other values more easily override the service ethic. British doctors have worked hard to defend the NHS, to retain the conditions in which they can practice medicine truly professionally. The majority of them have shared the general British belief that, while it is proper for health care workers to be decently rewarded for the difficult and skilled tasks which they perform, it is nevertheless obscene to make profit out of illness and suffering. There are limits to what any one doctor can do to control the conditions of her or his service, crucially important although they are. They are also to some extent outside the control of the profession as a whole. However, the new professionals will continue to limit damage which can be done by the profit motive and to work towards a situation in which they are able to offer a decent service to all who need it.

Bibliography

Note

References to General Medical Council (GMC) *Annual Reports* and *Minutes* (pub: GMC, London) are cited in the text. *Annual Reports* have sometimes been published in the year to which they refer and sometimes in the subsequent year. To avoid confusion they are cited throughout as *GMC Annual Report for* [year]. *Minutes* are dated by the year to which they refer. Their volume numbers are cited in roman numerals.

Alderson, D.P. (1988). *Choosing for Children: Parents' Consent to Surgery*, Oxford, Oxford University Press, reprinted (1990), Oxford, Oxford University Press.

Anon. (1989). 'Unbelievable happenings a painful reality', *British Medical Journal*, **299**: 401.

Anwar, M. and Ali, A. (1987). *Overseas Doctors: Experience and Expectations*, Commission for Racial Equality, London.

Arney, W.R. (1982). *Power and the Profession of Obstetrics*, University of Chicago Press, Chicago and London.

ASCHCEW (1989). NHS *Complaints Procedure: a Report of a Conference held 11/10/88*, Health News Briefing, Association of Community Health Councils for England & Wales, London.

Bhattacharya, S.C. (1983). 'The origins and early work of the GMC', in *GMC Annual Report for 1982*, GMC, London.

Bolt, D., Robertson, R. F., Williams, D. I., Walton, J. and Yellowlees, H. (1989). *British Medical Journal*, *298*, p. 1641.

British Medical Association (1973). 'BMA's evidence to the Merrison Inquiry', *British Medical Journal*, Supplement, no. 3651, 159–175.

Bynum, W.F. and Porter, R. (eds) (1987). *Medical Fringe and Medical Orthodoxy 1750–1850*, Croom Helm, London.

Campbell, D. (1989). 'An investigative journalist looks at medical ethics', *British Medical Journal*, **298**: 1171.

Clark, A. (1968). *Working Life of Women in the Seventeenth Century* (1st edn 1919), Frank Cass, London.

Crisp, A. (1983). *GMC Annual Report for 1982*, p. 32.

Crisp, A. (1988). 'Medical education', *GMC Annual Report for 1987*, GMC, London.

Davies Report (1973). *Report of the Committee on Hospital Complaints Procedure*, DHSS, London.

DHSS (1972). *Management Arrangements for the Reorganized NHS*, DHSS, London.

Donnison, J. (1988). *Midwives and Medical Men: A History of Inter-Professional Rivalry and Women's Rights,* 2nd edn, Historical Publications, New Barnett.

Dowie, R. (1987). *Postgraduate Medical Education and Training: the System in England and Wales,* King Edwards Hospital Fund for London, London.

Draper, M.R. (1978). 'European Economic Community: the first year's experience of free movement of doctors', *GMC Annual Report for 1977,* GMC, London, pp. 20–22.

Draper, M.R. (1983). 'The GMC from 1950 to 1982: a Registrar's impression', *GMC Annual Report for 1982,* GMC, London.

Fisher, N. and Fahy, T. (1990). 'Sexual relations between doctors and patients', *Journal of the Royal Society of Medicine,* **83**: 681–683.

GMC (1957). *Recommendations on Basic Medical Education,* GMC, London.

GMC (1967). *Recommendations on Basic Medical Education,* GMC, London.

GMC (1976). *Professional Conduct and Discipline,* GMC, London.

GMC (1977). *Survey of Basic Medical Education,* GMC, London.

GMC (1979). *Professional Conduct and Discipline,* GMC, London.

GMC (1980). *Recommendations on Basic Medical Education,* GMC, London.

GMC (1981). *Professional Conduct and Discipline: Fitness to Practise,* GMC, London.

GMC (1983). *Professional Conduct and Discipline: Fitness to Practise,* GMC, London.

GMC (1987a). *Recommendations on the Training of Specialists,* GMC London.

GMC (1987b). *Recommendations on General Clinical Training,* GMC, London.

GMC (1989). *Professional Conduct and Discipline: Fitness to Practise,* GMC, London.

GMC (1991). *Professional Conduct and Discipline: Fitness to Practise,* GMC, London.

Gillon, R. (1990). 'Professional ethics: on transmitting complaints to colleagues', *Journal of Medical Ethics,* **3**: 115.

Green, D. (1985). *Which Doctor? a Critical Analysis of the Professional Barriers to Competition in Health Care,* Institute of Economic Affairs, London.

Gullick, D. (1980). 'The general medical steeple chase', *World Medicine,* **15**, 12: 79–84.

Ham, C., Dingwall, R., Fenn, P. and Harris, D. (1988). *Medical Negligence: Compensation and Accountability,* Kings Fund Institute, London.

Havard, J.D.J. (1989a). *Medical Negligence: the Mounting Dilemma.* The Stevens Lecture for the laity, Royal Society of Medicine, London.

Havard, J. (1989b). 'Advertising by doctors and the public interest', *British Medical Journal,* **298**: 903.

Hill, D. (1975). 'Complaints against doctors', *GMC Annual Report for 1974,* GMC, London.

HMSO (1987). *Promoting Better Health,* the government's programme for improving primary health care', Cm. 249, HMSO, London.

HMSO (1988). *Review of Restrictive Trade Practices: a Consultative Document,* Cm. 331, HMSO, London.

HMSO (1989a). *Working for Patients,* Cm. 555, HMSO, London.

HMSO (1989b). *Services of Medical Practitioners,* Monopolies and Mergers Commission, Cm. 582, HMSO, London.

Hoffenberg, R. (1987). *Clinical Freedom,* The Rock Carling Fellowship, 1986, The Nuffield Provincial Hospitals Trust, London.

Horder, J., Ennis, J., Hirsch, S., Laurence, D., Marinker, M., Murray, D., Wakeling, A., Yudkin, J.S. (1984). 'An important opportunity: an open letter to the GMC', *British Medical Journal,* **288**: 1507–1511.

Irvine, D. (1991). 'The advertising of doctors' services', *Journal of Medical Ethics,* **17**: 35–40.

Jefferys, M. and Sachs, H. (1983). *Rethinking General Practice: Dilemmas in Primary Medical Care,* Tavistock, London.

Kennedy, I. (1983). *The Unmasking of Medicine* Granada, London.

Kennedy, I. (1987). 'Review of the year 2: confidentiality, competence and malpractice', in *Medicine in Contemporary Society: King's College Studies 1986–7* (ed. P. Byrne), King Edward's Hospital Fund for London. London.

Kilpatrick, R. (1985). 'Inspecting, by the inspected', *GMC Annual Report for 1984,* GMC, London.

Kilpatrick, R. (1989a). 'Profile of the GMC: portrait or caricature?' *British Medical Journal,* **299**: 109–112.

Kilpatrick, R. (1989b). 'Medical Education', *GMC Annual Report for 1988,* GMC, London.

Klein, R. (1973). *Complaints against Doctors: a study in professional accountability,* Charles Knight, London.

Klein, R. and Shinebourne, A. (1972). 'Doctors' discipline', *New Society,* **22**, 528: 399–401.

Larkin, G. (1983). *Occupational Monopoly and Modern Medicine,* Tavistock, London and New York.

Larson, M. S. (1977). *The Rise of Professionalism: a sociological analysis,* University of California Press, Berkeley, Los Angeles, London.

Lock, S. (1989). 'Regulating Doctors', *British Medical Journal,* **299**: 137–138.

Loudon, I. (1986). *Medical Care and the General Practitioner 1750–1850,* Clarendon Press, Oxford.

McCallum, A. (1989). 'First Impressions', *GMC Annual Report for 1989,* GMC, London.

Macdonald, K. (1989). 'Building Respectability', *Sociology,* 23, 1, pp. 55–80.

McManus *et al.* (1977). 'The preregistration year: chaos by consensus', *Lancet,* **i**: 413–417.

Merrison Report (1975). *Report of the Committee of Inquiry into the Regulation of the Medical Profession,* Cmnd. 6018, HMSO, London.

Oakley, A. (1976). 'Wise woman and medicine man: changes in the management of childbirth', in *The Rights and Wrongs of Women* (eds J. Mitchell and A. Oakley), Harmondsworth, Penguin.

Palermo, G. B. (1990). 'On psycho-therapist–patient sex: discussion paper', *Journal of the Royal Society of Medicine,* **83**: 715–719.

Paxman, J. (1991). *Friends in High Places: Who Runs Britain?* Harmondsworth, Penguin.

Pelling, M. (1987). 'Medical practice in the early modern period: trade or profession?', in *The Professions in Early Modern England* (ed. W. Prest), Croom Helm, London.

Peterson, M.J. (1978). *The Medical Profession in Mid-Victorian London,* University of California Press, Berkeley, California.

Porter, R. (1982). *English Society in the Eighteenth Century,* Penguin, Harmondsworth.

Porter, R. (1987). *Disease, Medicine and Society in England 1550–1860,* Macmillan Educational, Basingstoke.

Pyke-Lees, W. (1958). *Centenary of the GMC 1858–1958: The History and Present Work of the Council,* GMC, London.

Rhodes, P. (1989). *British Medical Journal,* **298**: 1641.

Richardson, Lord (1980). 'The metamorphosis of the Council', *GMC Annual Report for 1979,* GMC, London.

Richardson, Lord (1983). 'The Council transformed', *GMC Annual Report for 1982*, GMC, London.

Robinson, J. (1988). *A Patient Voice at the GMC: a Lay Member's View of the GMC, Health Rights*, Report 1, Health Rights, London.

Rosenthal, M. M. (1987). *Dealing with Medical Malpractice*, Tavistock, London.

Scott, J. (1984). 'Women and the GMC', *British Medical Journal*, **289**: 1764–1767.

Scott, J. (1988). 'Women and the GMC: the struggle for representation', *Journal of the Royal Society of Medicine*, Vol. 81, 164–166.

Shaw (1989). 'Medical Education', *GMC Annual Report for 1989*, GMC, London.

Simanowitz, A. (1990). 'How to call the medical profession to account?' Paper presented to RSM/BMA Conference on Medical Standards, Peer Review, Audit and Accountability. London: Association for the Victims of Medical Accidents. Mimeo.

Smith, D. (1987). *The Everyday World as Problematic*. The Open University Press, Milton Keynes.

Smith, D. J. (1980). *Overseas Doctors in the National Health Service*, Policy Studies Institute, London.

Smith, R. (1989a). 'Doctors, unethical treatments and turning a blind eye', *British Medical Journal*, **298**: 1125–1126.

Smith, R. (1989b). 'The day of judgement comes closer', *British Medical Journal*, **298**: 1241–1244.

Smith, R. (1989c). '1978 and all that', *British Medical Journal*, **298**: 1297–1300.

Smith, R. (1989d). 'Medical education and the GMC: controlled or stifled?' *British Medical Journal*, **298**: 1372–1375.

Smith, R. (1989e). 'Overseas doctors: diminishing controversy', *British Medical Journal*, **298**: 1441–1444.

Smith, R. (1989f). 'Discipline I: the hordes at the gates', *British Medical Journal*, **298**: 1502–1505.

Smith, R. (1989g). 'Discipline II: the preliminary screener–a powerful gatekeeper', *British Medical Journal*, **298**: 1569–1571.

Smith, R. (1989h). 'Discipline III: the final stages', *British Medical Journal*, **298**: 1632–1634.

Smith, R. (1989i). 'Dealing with sickness and incompetence: success and failure', *British Medical Journal*, **298**: 1695–1698.

Smith, R. (1989j). 'The council's internal problems', *British Medical Journal*, **299**: 40–43.

Stacey, F. (1975). *British Government 1966–1975 Years of Reform*, Oxford University Press, London.

Stacey, M. (1988a). *The Sociology of Health and Healing: a Textbook*, Unwin Hyman, London.

Stacey, M. (1988b). 'The GMC: public protection and professional unity', *ESRC Newsletter*, **62**: 25–26.

Stacey, M. (1989a). 'The GMC and professional accountability' (A revised version of the Frank Stacey Memorial Lecture of 1986) *Public Policy and Administration*, **4**, 1: 12–27.

Stacey, M. (1989b). 'A Sociologist Looks at the GMC', *Lancet* (i) April 1: 713–714.

Stacey, M. (1990). 'The British GMC and Medical Ethics'. In *Social Science Perspectives on Medical Ethics* (ed. G. Weisz), Kluwer Academic Publications, Dordrecht; reprinted in paperback, University of Pennsylvania Press, Philadelphia, 1991.

Stacey, M. (1991). 'Medical accountability: a background paper', in *The 1991 Annual*

Volume: Centre of Medical Law and Ethics, King's College, London; John Wiley, Chichester.

Stacey, M. (forthcoming, 1992). 'A sociologist in action', *Sociology in Action* (ed. G. Payne and M. Cross), Macmillan, London.

Stimson, G. and Webb, B. (1975). *Going to see the Doctor: the consultation process in general practice*, Routledge and Kegan Paul, London and Boston.

Todd Report (1968). *Report of the Royal Commission on Medical Education*, Cmnd. 3569, HMSO, London.

Waddington, I. (1984). *The Medical Profession in the Industrial Revolution*, Gill and Macmillan, London.

Walton, J. (1979). 'The Council and the pre-registration year', *GMC Annual Report for 1978*, GMC, London.

Walton, J. (1982). *GMC Annual Report for 1981*, GMC, London.

Watkins, S. (1987). *Medicine and Labour: the Politics of a Profession*, Lawrence and Wishart, London.

Williams, D.I. (1988). 'Registration of overseas qualified doctors', *GMC Annual Report for 1987*, GMC, London.

Wilson, E. (1990). *Hallucinations: Life in the Post-modern City*, Hutchinson Radius, London.

Wood, D. (1987). 'On reflection: 1969–86', *GMC Annual Report for 1986*, GMC, London, pp. 7–9.

Wright, R. (1980). 'Registration of overseas qualified doctors', *GMC Annual Report for 1979*, GMC, London.

Index

Note: page numbers in *italics* refer to figures and tables

Index compiled by Jill Halliday